Health Statistics

HEALTH AFFAIRS INFORMATION GUIDE SERIES

Series Editor: Winifred Sewell, Health Science Information Consultant, currently associated with the University of Maryland and the National Health Planning Information Center

Also in this series:

BIOETHICS—*Edited by Doris Goldstein**

CROSS-NATIONAL STUDY OF HEALTH SYSTEMS: CONCEPTS, METHODS, AND DATA SOURCES—*Edited by Ray H. Elling*

CROSS-NATIONAL STUDY OF HEALTH SYSTEMS BY COUNTRY AND WORLD REGIONS—*Edited by Ray H. Elling**

EDUCATION IN THE HEALTH PROFESSIONS—*Edited by Elizabeth A. Martinsen**

HEALTH CARE ADMINISTRATION—*Edited by Dwight A. Morris and Lynne Darby Morris*

HEALTH CARE COSTS AND FINANCING—*Edited by Rita Keintz**

HEALTH CARE POLITICS, POLICY, AND LEGISLATION—*Edited by Joel M. Lee**

HEALTH MAINTENANCE THROUGH FOOD AND NUTRITION—*Edited by Helen Ullrich**

HEALTH PLANNING—*Edited by Lewis Lefko**

HEALTH SCIENCES AUDIOVISUALS—*Edited by Laura P. Barrett**

HUMAN ECOLOGY—*Edited by Frederick Sargent II**

INTERFACE OF MEDICINE AND THE LAW—*Edited by Sal Fiscina, James Zimmerly, Paul Connors, and Janet B. Seifert**

MEDICAL INFORMATION TRANSFER—*Edited by Winifred Sewell and Marie Dickerman**

THE PROFESSIONAL AND SCIENTIFIC LITERATURE ON PATIENT EDUCATION—*Edited by Lawrence W. Green and Connie C. Kansler**

QUALITY MAINTENANCE AND EVALUATION OF HEALTH CARE—*Edited by Jay Glasser and Irene Eastling**

SURVEY OF EMERGENCY MEDICAL SERVICES SYSTEM RESOURCES—*Edited by Carlos Fernandez-Caballero and Marianne Fernandez-Caballero**

THERAPEUTIC MATERIALS IN THE HEALTH SYSTEM—*Edited by Winifred Sewell and Marie Dickerman**

*in preparation

The above series is part of the
GALE INFORMATION GUIDE LIBRARY

The Library consists of a number of separate series of guides covering major areas in the social sciences, humanities, and current affairs.

General Editor: Paul Wasserman, Professor and former Dean, School of Library and Information Services, University of Maryland

Managing Editor: Denise Allard Adzigian, Gale Research Company

Health Statistics

A GUIDE TO INFORMATION SOURCES

Volume 4 in the Health Affairs Information Guide Series

Frieda O. Weise

Head, Public Services Unit
Reference Section
National Library of Medicine
Bethesda, Maryland

Gale Research Company
Book Tower, Detroit, Michigan 48226

Copyright © 1980 by
Frieda O. Weise

ISBN 0-8103-1412-6
Library of Congress Catalog Card Number 80-12039

No part of this book may be reproduced in any form without permission in writing from the publisher, except by a reviewer who wishes to quote brief passages or entries in connection with a review written for inclusion in a magazine or newspaper. Manufactured in the United States of America.

VITA

Frieda O. Weise is currently head, Public Services Unit, Reference Section, at the National Library of Medicine, Bethesda, Maryland. She received an A.M.L.S. from the University of Michigan in 1973 and her B.A. in history from Albright College, Reading, Pennsylvania, in 1964. She is a member of the Medical Library Association and the District of Columbia Library Association. She is also an instructor for the continuing education course, Statistical Sources for Health Sciences Librarians, for the Medical Library Association.

CONTENTS

Foreword	ix
Preface	xiii
Introduction	xv
Abbreviations	xvii

Chapter 1. General References	1
Textbooks	1
Directories	4
Dictionaries and Handbooks	7
Catalogs	8
Bibliographies	10
Indexes and Abstracting Services	14
Machine-Readable Files	17
Guides to Machine-Readable Files	18
Data Files	19
Bibliographic Files	20
Compilations of Health Statistics	22
Vital and Health Statistics Series	22
General Compilations	24
Chapter 2. Vital Statistics	31
Chapter 3. Morbidity	37
Series	37
Specific Diseases and Health Conditions	38
Accidents and Injuries	39
Alcoholism	39
Botulism	40
Cancer	40
Diabetes	43
Disability	43
Drug Abuse	44
Epilepsy	45
Heart Disease	46
Hypertension	46
Mental Health	46

Contents

Nutrition	47
Occupational Health	47
Smoking	48
Tuberculosis	48
Venereal Disease	49
Vision and Hearing	49
Miscellaneous	50
Chapter 4. Health Resources	53
Health Facilities	53
Health Manpower	55
Health Education	62
Chapter 5. Health Services Utilization	65
Chapter 6. Health Care Costs and Expenditures	71
Chapter 7. Population Characteristics	79
Appendix A. Newsletters and Journals	83
Newsletters	83
Journals	84
Appendix B. Government Agencies	87
State Agencies	87
Federal Agencies	92
International Agencies	95
Appendix C. Associations	97
Appendix D. Regional Depository Libraries	101
Appendix E. Suppliers of Bibliographic Data Files	105
Glossary	107
Author Index	111
Title Index	115
Subject Index	123

FOREWORD

Interest in health and the resources and activities that make it possible is not new. However, the concepts of health as a national resource and as a human right have emerged in the recent past. Legislation during the last two decades has led from these concepts to a complex system with some unsurprising growing pains.

Many people have come into the field, bringing a multiplicity of backgrounds to supplement the traditional health sciences. In addition, today's laymen must make decisions on health care at all levels--from voting for or against legislators who will shape health laws, through serving on local health planning boards, to becoming participants in informed decisions on their own health care. The new recruits and the laymen have in common the need for all kinds of information on social, business, legal, ethical, and other aspects of medicine.

Much of this information has previously been unavailable and not readily understandable to the new audiences. Attempts to satisfy the need have resulted in burgeoning publications on a variety of subjects ranging from the broad to the specific. These new publications are in many forms; from carefully edited, important texts to poorly conceived and executed technical reports, with a vast array in between. There are journals, newsletters, association and university guidebooks and models, statistical reports, and audiovisuals--all of varying quality and format.

Several problems have resulted. In the first place, there has not yet emerged a major bibliographic resource, such as the National Library of Medicine and Excerpta Medica provide for the clinical and research aspects of medicine. In addition, some of the novices in the field are not accustomed to using published literature in any form, let alone the complex of primary, secondary, and tertiary publications with which their counterparts in clinical medicine and research have become familiar.

It is the purpose of the Health Affairs Series in the Gale Information Guide Library to provide a guide for all participants in the complex health care system to information on the system itself--on the process of the delivery of health

Foreword

care. We are concerned with the management of the system and with how researchers, educators, and practitioners assure the best health possible to each individual. We are not concerned with the content of the information with which the researcher, educator, or practitioner deals, but rather with his mode of functioning in a real world of people with different racial, ethnic, sexual, financial, and geographic backgrounds. For example, we are not interested in how a surgical procedure is carried out, but we are concerned with its availability to those who need it. If one understands the social sciences broadly, then the Health Affairs Series covers the social aspects of medicine.

Among those social aspects we include ones which are focused on the individual in relation to his environment, his education for full participation in his own health care, and his social, political, legal, and ethical responsibilities. In addition, we include all components involved with providing facilities and resources necessary for health care delivery. Individual volumes cover: health statistics; human ecology--both man-environment interactions and manipulations and their outcomes and intervention strategies; health maintenance through food and nutrition; the professional and scientific literature of patient education; health care politics, policy, and legislation; cross-national study of health systems; health planning; health care costs and financing; quality maintenance and evaluation of health care; health care administration; emergency medical service systems; preventive, diagnostic, and therapeutic materials in the health system; education in the health professions; medical information transfer; bioethics; and interface of medicine and the law.

Thus, just as the Gale Information Guide Library encompasses a broad spectrum of all fields of knowledge, the Health Affairs Series endeavors to be comprehensive with respect to the social aspects of medicine.

The user may ask, "Why another bibliography when there are already so many?" We agree, but the Health Affairs guides are much more then bibliographies. All contain a careful selection of materials for the intended audience, an evaluation of these materials in annotations and introductory paragraphs, and directions for finding further information. There are lists of many sources of information, such as information centers, schools, publishers, and audiovisuals. The journals which one should read regularly to keep up with the field are mentioned and annotated. In short, the reader will find specific resources as they are developed.

Because all of the social sciences dealing with health affairs are interrelated, it is both impossible and undesirable to prescribe strict limits for each individual volume, excluding from one anything included in another. Instead, each volume of the series is complete for the individual who is interested in only one specific subject. At the same time, other volumes serve as excellent supplements when the user wishes to go into related topics in greater depth.

Foreword

A person interested in any of the social aspects of medicine should be able to find a volume that focuses on that interest, although the depth of coverage will vary with the topic. In some instances the amount of literature available determined the division of the series into specific volumes, and coverage of materials is highly selective; in other cases, the choice of volume topic was somewhat arbitrary, determined by the independence which may have allowed for greater depth of coverage of a topic. The series editor takes responsibility for the general organization and coverage of a topic. The series editor takes responsibility for the general organization and coverage of the series, but has left to the judgement of the volume editors decisions on individual items to be included or excluded. The series should thus be helpful to the user not only for what he is able to find in the individual volumes, but for how it has been sifted to exclude those materials that would send him down blind alleys.

We hope that our audience for the series will consist of newcomers to the fields involved, as well as researchers and practitioners who have worked with health affairs in the past but need to renew their familiarity with resources in some aspect of their major current interests. We hope especially that the guides will be useful in the education of students who have chosen one or more of the fields covered for their future careers. And finally, we have tried to make the volumes simple and direct enough that they will provide the informed layperson with access to the information resources needed to make decisions about future procedures and policies in assurance of the best match between national resources and the health care of the nation.

The need for an up-to-date bibliography of statistical resources for the health sciences is expressed very frequently. The requirement for data upon which to make decisions is both urgent and changing, and new health measures are constantly being developed. In such a dynamic field, the task of preparing a bibliography of sources of health statistics is not an easy one.

In the following bibliography, Frieda Weise has developed a straightforward analysis of the myriad of sources and presented them directly and simply, in a manner which satisfies these needs. In her introductions to chapters, she suggests where further resources should be created. In short, she has accomplished the challenging objective of providing a guide to statistical data for the health scientist and librarian which will serve current needs and point the user in the direction of future resources.

Winifred Sewell, Series Editor
Cabin John, Maryland

PREFACE

The purpose of this volume is to present the librarian, the information professional, the student, and the health professional with a guide to the basic sources of vital and health statistics in the United States. Vital and health statistics are defined broadly here to include the following subjects:

   natality and mortality
   marriage and divorce
   morbidity
   health care facilities
   health manpower
   health services utilization
   health care costs and expenditures
   health professions education
   population characteristics

In determining the criteria for inclusion in this bibliography, the peculiarities of health data collection in the United States weighed heavily. The larger part of the sources cited are government publications since the majority of the vital and health statistics are gathered by the local, state, or federal government. Private health organizations and professional associations also figure prominently in the collection and publication of health statistics. For the most part, journal articles concerning vital or health statistics were not included since this information is limited in scope, is quickly out of date, and can be accessed more efficiently through current indexes, abstracts, or computerized data bases.

Chapter 1 provides general references whose scope is quite broad while chapters 2-7 contain references to publications specific to the subject of the chapter. Chapter 2 covers vital statistics; chapter 3 covers morbidity data for both communicable and chronic diseases. Chapter 4 presents references pertaining to health resources data and chapters 5 and 6 cover health services utilization and health care costs and expenditures. The final chapter cites references to population data.

The appendixes include newsletters and journals as well as lists of private associations, government agencies, and libraries from which either data or publications may be obtained.

INTRODUCTION

Vital and health statistics information is essential to the delivery of health care in the United States. It has often been said that statistics are the eyes and ears of the health planner, epidemiologist, and health professional. With the passage of the National Health Planning and Resources Development Act of 1974 (Public Law 93-641), this has been made more than abundantly clear.

The act established local health systems agencies (HSAs) throughout the country to improve the health of the residents in the health service area covered by the HSA. To meet this responsibility the health systems agency must assemble and analyze data concerning the health of the area's residents, as well as its health care delivery system, health resources, utilization of health resources, and even environmental factors affecting long-term health conditions. It is to utilize existing data whenever possible. Those who are users of health data therefore include a wide range of public and private agencies, organizations, and individuals concerned with planning, provision, or evaluation of health services and health resources.

Clearly the need for vital and health statistics data is growing with increased health planning efforts. However, can it be said that existing data provide the information needed to those who are expected to use them to fulfill their goals? The U.S. Department of Health, Education, and Welfare in its HEALTH STATISTICS PLAN, FISCAL YEAR 1976-77, aptly answers this in the following statement:

> Health statistics production in this country presents a picture of uncoordinated data collection, aggregation, presentation and analysis among various Federal, State, local and non-governmental sources. The separate efforts underway are frequently duplicative of one another and despite common goals, possess little of the continuity, compatibility and standardization which are essential to a reliable health statistics system . . . [1]

---

1. U.S. Department of Health, Education, and Welfare, HEALTH STATISTICS PLAN, FISCAL YEAR 1976-77 (Washington, D.C.: Government Printing Office, 1975), p. 20.

Introduction

This evaluation was affirmed in a study of health data and health data systems done by the Office of Technology Assessment in January 1977. The study stated that "there is a plethora of uncoordinated and expensive health data systems," that there is no authority either in the federal government or the private health industry to define and promote compatibility among health care collection systems, and that there is no defined core data set. In short, health data affairs are in a "chaotic" state.[2]

This is not terribly encouraging for the users of health data. Users include many others in addition to health planners already mentioned. They can range from the student writing a paper, to the epidemiologist interested in the etiology of disease, to a senator debating health policy in Congress.

Librarians and other information professionals who are intermediaries in the search for health data have found it a most frustrating subject. Available data are varied in coverage, completeness, and uniformity. Health data are collected by government agencies, private associations, and voluntary organizations. The search can be endless and in the end fruitless.

It is hoped that this bibliography will shed some light on the availability of vital and health statistics data for a variety of users. The introductory remarks for each chapter briefly discuss gaps in the data for the particular subject covered. The selected bibliographies represent the best currently available (and in many cases only available) materials for the subject.

---

2. David R. Hutchinson, "The Office of Technology Assessment Health Data Study: A Preliminary Report," HEALTH SERVICES RESEARCH 13, no. 2 (1978): 103-10.

ABBREVIATIONS

AAMC	American Association of Medical Colleges
ADM	Alcohol, Drug Abuse and Mental Health Administration
AHA	American Hospital Association
AHEC	Area Health Education Center
APA	American Psychiatric Association
APHA	American Public Health Association
BHRD	Bureau of Health Resources Development
BLS	Bureau of Labor Statistics
CDC	Center for Disease Control
CPHA	Commission on Professional and Hospital Activities
FAO	Food and Agricultural Organization
FDA	Food and Drug Administration
FNG	Foreign Nurse Graduates
HRA	Health Resources Administration
HSA	Health Systems Agency
IARC	International Agency for Research on Cancer
LPN	Licensed Practical Nurse
NCES	National Center for Education Statistics
NCHS	National Center for Health Statistics
NEISS	National Electronic Injury Surveillance System
NHPIC	National Health Planning Information Center
NIDA	National Institute of Drug Abuse
NIH	National Institutes of Health
NIMH	National Institute of Mental Health

Abbreviations

NINCDS	National Institute of Neurological, Communicative Disorders and Stroke
PAHO	Pan-American Health Organization
PAS	Professional Activity Study of the Commission on Professional and Hospital Activities
PSRO	Professional Standards Review Organization
SMSA	Standard Metropolitan Statistical Area
SSA	Social Security Administration
UNESCO	United Nations Educational, Social, and Cultural Organization
WHO	World Health Organization

Chapter 1
GENERAL REFERENCES

This chapter is intended to provide the reader with references to general sources of information on health statistics. The sources are organized by the following formats: Textbooks, Directories, Dictionaries and Handbooks, Catalogs, Bibliographies, Indexes and Abstracting Services, Machine-Readable Files, and Compilations of Health Statistics.

TEXTBOOKS

This section includes a selection of textbooks which introduce the reader to the nature and uses of epidemiology and health statistics. Especially useful for the beginner is the HANDBOOK OF COMMUNITY HEALTH (see no. 1.7).

1.1 Alderson, Michael. AN INTRODUCTION TO EPIDEMIOLOGY. New York: Macmillan, 1976.

   Describes various approaches of epidemiology with special emphasis on study design. Discusses use of cross-sectional, retrospective, and prospective studies and their advantages and disadvantages, as well as intervention studies, including preventive, clinical and medical-care trials. Also discusses mortality and morbidity statistics and their uses.

1.2 Barker, D.J.P. PRACTICAL EPIDEMIOLOGY. New York: Churchill Livingstone, 1976.

   A short, practical manual for students and health professionals in developing countries. Includes discussion of the sequence of an epidemiological study and describes the investigation of epidemics and trials of preventive measures as well.

1.3 Bourke, Geoffrey J., and McGilvray, James. INTERPRETATION AND USES OF MEDICAL STATISTICS. 2d ed. Oxford, Engl.: Blackwell Scientific Publications, 1975.

   Emphasis on the interpretation of medical statistics. Designed to aid graduates and undergraduates in their understanding of

General References

statistics as applied to medicine and allied subjects. Definitions of terms and examples throughout.

1.4 Burton, Lloyd Edward, and Smith, Hugh Hollingsworth. PUBLIC HEALTH AND COMMUNITY MEDICINE FOR THE ALLIED MEDICAL PROFESSIONS. 2d ed. Baltimore, Md.: Williams and Wilkins, 1975.

Offers a thorough discussion of epidemiology, its uses, and methods in chapter 4, "The Methodology of Public Health." Covers uses and methods of vital and demographic statistics, as well, with many examples.

1.5 Duncan, Robert C., et al. INTRODUCTORY BIOSTATISTICS FOR HEALTH SCIENCES. New York: Wiley, 1977.

Intended to enable health science professionals to apply basic descriptive and inferential statistical techniques to their field. Requires elementary background in algebra. Chapters divided into sections: Overview, Objectives, Foundations, Methodology, and Problems.

1.6 Friedman, Gary D. PRIMER OF EPIDEMIOLOGY. New York: McGraw-Hill, 1974.

Textbook for medical students and health care professionals who need a basic understanding of epidemiological terms, methods, and types of studies. Stresses practical usefulness of epidemiology and presents a general guide for conducting an epidemiological investigation.

1.7 Grant, Murray. HANDBOOK OF COMMUNITY HEALTH. 2d ed. Philadelphia: Lea Febiger, 1975.

Presents the basics of public health and preventive medicine. Chapter 1 on epidemiology and chapter 2 on health statistics provide concise information concerning the uses and importance of both to the health care field. Gives definitions and examples of types of health statistics and epidemiological studies as well.

1.8 Hill, Sir Austin Bradford. A SHORT TEXTBOOK OF MEDICAL STATISTICS. London: Hodder and Stoughton, 1977.

Detailed discussion of the methods of collection of statistics and their presentation. Presents problems involved in sampling techniques and interpretation of data. Covers correlation and regression, calculation of the correlation coefficient, standardized death rates and indexes, life tables, and measures of morbidity, as well as clinical trials.

General References

1.9   Kilpatrick, S. James. STATISTICAL PRINCIPLES IN HEALTH CARE INFORMATION. Baltimore, Md.: University Park Press, 1973.

   Basic introduction for the nonmathematician. Includes chapters on the nature, collection, and interpretation of health care data; on epidemiology and the design of surveys; and on statistical concepts such as probability, distributions, and significance.

1.10 Lancaster, H.O. AN INTRODUCTION TO MEDICAL STATISTICS. New York: Wiley, 1974.

   Provides an elementary review of vital statistics and the application of statistical methods to clinical and laboratory medicine. Chapters on death rates, theory of life table construction, and fertility rates.

1.11 Lilienfeld, Abraham M. FOUNDATIONS OF EPIDEMIOLOGY. New York: Oxford University Press, 1976.

   An introductory presentation to the concepts and methods of epidemiology as they apply to disease. Emphasis on aspects of epidemiological reasoning as it derives inferences about the etiology of disease from population data.

1.12 Lowe, C.R., and Livanga, S.K. HEALTH STATISTICS: A MANUAL FOR TEACHERS OF MEDICAL STUDENTS. Handbooks sponsored by the IEA and WHO, no. 1. Oxford, Engl.: Oxford University Press, 1978.

   Describes ways in which health statistics are used by health practitioners; gives a list of health statistical knowledge and abilities which medical students should be taught; describes basic teaching techniques for the material; and gives objectives for the teaching of health statistics.

1.13 Phillips, David A. BASIC STATISTICS FOR HEALTH SCIENCE STUDENTS. San Francisco: W.H. Freeman and Co., 1978.

   Intended as a reference book for those with a background in statistics. Covers a wide variety of statistical techniques divided into two broad areas--descriptive and inferential. Contains exercises in chapters and answers at the end of the book.

1.14 Sartwell, Phillip E. PREVENTIVE MEDICINE AND PUBLIC HEALTH. 10th ed. New York: Appleton-Century-Crofts, 1973.

   Discusses measurements of health and disease, general epidemiology and the epidemiology of infections in the chapter on epidemiology. Includes uses and methods of prevalence surveys, surveillance of diseases, and cohort studies.

General References

1.15 Wilner, Daniel M., et al. INTRODUCTION TO PUBLIC HEALTH. 7th ed. New York: Macmillan, 1978.

> Presents a basic overview of demography, vital statistics, and epidemiology in chapter 10. Includes discussion of census collection and procedures, vital registration data, and vital statistics rates with definitions and examples for each. Also covers briefly the scope of epidemiology.

DIRECTORIES

The directories listed in this section provide access to names of both government and private agencies which collect, publish, or otherwise provide access to statistical information in health. Of special interest is the DIRECTORY OF GOVERNMENT DOCUMENT COLLECTIONS AND LIBRARIANS (see no. 1.16), since many statistical publications originate with government agencies and are available at depository libraries throughout the United States.

The MEDICAL AND HEALTH INFORMATION DIRECTORY (see no. 1.19) describes a wide range of public agencies and private organizations not found in other directories.

Appendixes B and C list specific state, federal, and private agencies which gather and disseminate health statistics and appendix D lists the regional depository libraries in the United States.

1.16 American Library Association. Government Documents Round Table. DIRECTORY OF GOVERNMENT DOCUMENT COLLECTIONS AND LIBRARIANS. 2d ed. Washington, D.C.: Congressional Information Service, 1978.

> Provides a full range of information about government documents collections. Lists each library in geo-alphabetical order by state, city, and institution in the main entry section. Information includes the address, categories of documents collected, depository status, staff, and notes concerning access. Indexed by library staff.

1.17 ENCYCLOPEDIA OF ASSOCIATIONS. 13th ed. 3 vols. Edited by Nancy Yakes and Denise Akey. Detroit: Gale Research Co., 1979.

> Guide to national and international organizations which includes a section on medical and health organizations. Lists the address, telephone number, function, publications, number of members, founding date, committees, and annual meetings for each organization.

General References

1.18 International Agency for Research on Cancer. DIRECTORY OF ON-GOING RESEARCH ON CANCER EPIDEMIOLOGY. IARC Scientific Publication no. 17. Lyon, France: 1977.

    Contains 905 projects from 70 countries in the field of cancer epidemiology. Arranges descriptions of projects alphabetically by county and city and numbers them sequentially by (1) serial number and date of receipt, (2) principal investigator, (3) address of principal investigator, (4) anatomical cancer sites, (5) study type. Also provides list of population-based cancer registries.

1.19 Kruzas, Anthony T., ed. MEDICAL AND HEALTH INFORMATION DIRECTORY: A GUIDE TO STATE, NATIONAL AND INTERNATIONAL ORGANIZATIONS, GOVERNMENT AGENCIES, EDUCATIONAL INSTITUTIONS, HOSPITALS, GRANT-AWARD SOURCES, HEALTH CARE DELIVERY AGENCIES, JOURNALS, NEWSLETTERS, REVIEW SERIALS, ABSTRACTING SERVICES, PUBLISHERS, RESEARCH CENTERS, COMPUTERIZED DATA BANKS, AUDIOVISUAL SERVICES, AND LIBRARIES AND INFORMATION CENTERS. Detroit: Gale Research Co., 1977.

    Includes listings by federal and state departments and agencies, Health Systems Agencies (HSA), Poison Control Centers, Area Health Education Centers (AHEC), and MEDLINE Centers, all of which can be sources of statistical information. Gives addresses and telephone numbers.

1.19a NATIONAL HEALTH DIRECTORY. Washington, D.C.: Science and Health Publications, 1978.

    A comprehensive directory of key information on health programs and legislation. Includes congressmen, major health committees in the Congress, federal health agency personnel, state health officials, and federal regional officials. Also includes officials in PSROs, Health Systems Agencies, and Medicare and Medicaid. Agency and name index.

1.20 U.S. Department of Health, Education, and Welfare. HEALTH STATISTICS PLAN: FISCAL YEAR 19--. Washington, D.C.: Government Printing Office, 1976-77-- . Annual.

    Annual report on HEW plan for health data activities and inventory of health data projects in progress or planned. Includes inventories from all components of HEW. Extensive appendix, listing the health data activities in the department with a brief description of each project. Includes a telephone number to contact in the description. In some cases, cites availability of data, published or otherwise.

General References

1.21　U.S. Office of Management and Budget. FEDERAL STATISTICAL DIRECTORY. Washington, D.C.: Government Printing Office, 1935-- . Irregular.

　　　Lists, by organizational units of each agency, the names, office, and telephone numbers of key persons in statistical programs.

1.22　_____. STATISTICAL SERVICES OF THE UNITED STATES GOVERNMENT. Rev. ed. Washington, D.C.: Government Printing Office, 1976.

　　　Describes the federal statistical system and presents brief descriptions of the main economic and social statistical series gathered. Also contains a brief statement of the statistical responsibilities of each agency and a list of principal statistical publications.

1.23　U.S. Office of the Federal Register. UNITED STATES GOVERNMENT MANUAL. Washington, D.C.: Government Printing Office, 1935-- . Annual.

　　　Official handbook of the federal government. Describes purposes and programs of agencies and provides addresses and telephone numbers.

1.24　Wasserman, Paul. HEALTH ORGANIZATIONS OF THE UNITED STATES, CANADA, AND INTERNATIONALLY. 4th ed. Ann Arbor, Mich.: Edwards Brothers, 1977.

　　　Includes unofficial and nongovernmental organizations in health and related fields. Designed to guide "health and medical personnel, librarians, public officials, businessmen and others . . ." Includes address, telephone number, membership, publications, library, and the general purpose of each organization.

1.25　Wasserman, Paul, and Bernero, Jacqueline, eds. STATISTICS SOURCES: A SUBJECT GUIDE TO DATA ON INDUSTRIAL, BUSINESS, SOCIAL, EDUCATIONAL, FINANCIAL AND OTHER TOPICS FOR THE UNITED STATES AND INTERNATIONALLY. 5th ed. Detroit: Gale Research Co., 1977.

　　　Includes a selected, annotated bibliography, and a dictionary of statistical sources arranged by subjects which include health and medical services, vital statistics, and various diseases.

1.26　Wright, Nancy D., and Allen, Gene P. THE NATIONAL DIRECTORY OF STATE AGENCIES, 1976-77. 2d ed. Washington, D.C.: Information Resources Press, 1976.

　　　Covers state agencies by function. Lists functional categories alphabetically under each category, and under the specific

General References

agency in each state that is responsible for it. Includes address, name of head, and telephone number for each. Categories of interest are: aging, alcoholism, drug abuse, handicapped, health, mental health, and occupational safety and health.

DICTIONARIES AND HANDBOOKS

There are a limited number of these works since much of this information is generally included in textbooks. However, there are several sources which are useful, particularly A DISCURSIVE DICTIONARY OF HEALTH CARE (see no. 1.31) and the HEALTH PLANNING GLOSSARY (see no. 1.27).

1.27 Comprehensive Health Planning Agency of Southeastern Wisconsin. HEALTH PLANNING GLOSSARY. HRP-0015134. Springfield, Va.: National Technical Information Service, 1976.

Identifies and defines approximately four hundred terms used in health planning literature. Has a separate section on statistical terms used in measuring health status, as well as other terms used in statistical publications.

1.28 Kendall, Maurice G., and Buckland, William R. A DICTIONARY OF STATISTICAL TERMS. 3d ed., rev. and enl. New York: Hafner Publishing Co., 1971.

Contains definitions of statistical terms in current use, whether considered desirable or not. Omits elementary terms. Is not specific to health statistics but statistics generally.

1.29 Oreglia, Anthony, et al. DATA ACQUISITION AND ANALYSIS HANDBOOK FOR HEALTH PLANNERS. 2 vols. Health Planning Information Series, no. 4. HRP-0200401-2. Springfield, Va.: National Technical Information Service, 1977.

Handbook on acquiring, analyzing, and using secondary health data with illustrative tables and calculations. Discusses data on population, socioeconomic and health status, health resources, and utilization of different types of facilities.

1.30 U.S. Bureau of Health Planning and Resources Development. GUIDE TO THE COLLECTION AND USE OF HEALTH EXPENDITURES AND UTILIZATION DATA FOR HEALTH PLANNING AGENCIES. Health Planning Information Series, no. 5. HRP-0200501. Springfield, Va.: National Technical Information Service, 1978.

Intended to provide local health planning agencies with a guide to developing health expenditures profiles for their areas. Includes a list of health expenditure studies by state, regional, county, and city areas. Also gives names and addresses of information sources.

# General References

1.31 U.S. Congress. House of Representatives. Committee on Interstate and Foreign Commerce. A DISCURSIVE DICTIONARY OF HEALTH CARE. 94th Cong., 2d sess. Washington, D.C.: Government Printing Office, 1976.

> Includes statistical terms from epidemiology, insurance, health services, health and welfare programs, health manpower, health planning, Medicare and Medicaid.

CATALOGS

There are no catalogs devoted exclusively to health statistics. However, the following short list provides access to many of the statistical publications of international, federal, and state agencies. Most useful in identifying federal publications is Andriot's GUIDE TO U.S. GOVERNMENT STATISTICS (see no. 1.32), although its currency is hampered by the frequent beginning and ceasing of federal publications.

1.32 Andriot, John L. GUIDE TO U.S. GOVERNMENT STATISTICS. 4th ed. McLean, Va.: Documents Index, 1973.

> Annotated guide to recurring U.S. government statistical publications. Contains a complete listing of titles in the major statistical numbered series. Arranged by departments and agencies, listing publications containing statistical data, with agency, subject, and title indexes. Includes frequency, availability, and Superintendent of Documents classification number.

1.33 BUREAU OF THE CENSUS CATALOG. Washington, D.C.: Government Printing Office, 1946-- . Quarterly, cumulated annually, with monthly supplements.

> Annotated list of all reports issued by the bureau. Includes subject or data finder guides published by the bureau. Since 1964, includes unpublished material such as computer tapes, data files, and special tabulations. Geographic and subject indexes.

1.34 CHECKLIST OF STATE PUBLICATIONS. Englewood, Colo.: Information Handling Services, 1977-- . Quarterly.

> Lists state publications in alphabetical order by state and in alphabetical order by agency and title. Contains state published checklists plus whatever else could be identified. Gives availability, address, and price. Selected documents can be purchased on microfiche from Information Handling Services. Author, date, agency, and subject indexes.

General References

1.35 INTERNATIONAL BIBLIOGRAPHY INFORMATION DOCUMENTATION (IBID). New York: R.R. Bowker, 1973-- . Quarterly.

Provides bibliographic information on the current publications of the UN organizations: FAO, PAHO, UNESCO, and WHO. Includes books, periodicals, microforms. Gives information on how to acquire material and a list of national distributors.

1.36 MONTHLY CATALOG OF U.S. GOVERNMENT PUBLICATIONS. Washington, D.C.: Government Printing Office, 1895-- .

Lists government publications from all branches of the federal government. Periodicals appear in a supplement issue. Organized by issuing body with several index approaches: author, subject, title, and agency publication number. Semiannual indexes.

1.37 MONTHLY CHECKLIST OF STATE PUBLICATIONS. Washington, D.C.: Exchange and Gift Division, Library of Congress, 1910-- .

Lists state publications received by the Library of Congress. Arranged by state and issuing agency. Gives full bibliographic information. Annual index for serial publications.

1.38 U.S. Bureau of the Census. BUREAU OF THE CENSUS CATALOG OF PUBLICATIONS, 1790-1972. Washington, D.C.: Government Printing Office, 1974.

A one-volume comprehensive historical bibliography of sources for bureau of the census statistics from 1790 to 1972, comprised of two catalogs: (1) the CATALOG OF U.S. CENSUS PUBLICATIONS, 1790-1945, lists all materials issued by the Census Bureau and its predecessor organizations starting with the first census report of 1790; (2) the CENSUS CATALOG OF PUBLICATIONS, 1946-1972 updates the historical publication and describes the reports issued 1946-72.

1.39 U.S. Department of Health, Education, and Welfare. PUBLICATIONS CATALOG. Washington, D.C.: Government Printing Office, 1978.

Cumulative catalog covering July 1976-December 1977. Uses Anglo-American Cataloging Rules and Library of Congress main entries. Format like that of the MONTHLY CATALOG OF GOVERNMENT PUBLICATIONS (see no. 1.36) with text and five indexes: author, title, subject, series and report number, and Superintendent of Documents classification number.

1.40 U.S. Health Resources Administration. CATALOG OF PUBLICATIONS. DHEW publication no. (HRA) 78-615. Rockville, Md.: 1978. Semiannual.

General References

Lists most publications since 1974 of HRA units (National Center for Health Statistics, National Center for Health Services Research, Bureau of Health Manpower, and Bureau of Health Planning and Resources Development). Gives a brief description of each and availability statement from the publishing agency, the Government Printing Office, or the National Technical Information Service.

1.41 U.S. National Center for Health Statistics. CATALOGUE OF PUBLI-CATIONS, 1962-71. DHEW publication no. (HRA) 74-1300. Hyattsville, Md.: 1973. 1972 Supplement, DHEW publication no. (HRA) 73-1306, 1973; 1973 Supplement, DHEW publication no. (HRA) 74-1307. Rockville, Md.: 1974.

Complete listing and brief description of the publications issued by NCHS, grouped by fifteen broad subject categories. The majority of the publications in the catalog are from the center's Vital and Health Statistics Series.

1.42 U.S. Social Security Administration. Office of Research on Statistics. RESEARCH PUBLICATIONS. Washington, D.C.: n.d. Annual.

Catalog which identifies and annotates research publications produced by the SSA, Office of Research and Statistics (ORS). Tells availability, source, and price. Covers retirement and retirement research and disability research.

BIBLIOGRAPHIES

There have been few bibliographies published which provide coverage of all aspects of health statistics. Generally health statistics have been included as a section in bibliographies dealing with other health topics. Presented here is a variety of topical bibliographies which include health statistics as well as bibliographies devoted exclusively to health statistics. The most useful to date of any bibliographic guide (aside from the AMERICAN STATISTICS INDEX, no. 1.61) is the National Center for Health Statistics' FACTS AT YOUR FINGERTIPS (see no. 1.57). Another is SELECTED NATIONAL DATA SOURCES FOR HEALTH PLANNERS (see no. 1.50).

1.43 Ackroyd, Ted J., ed. HEALTH AND MEDICAL ECONOMICS: A GUIDE TO INFORMATION SOURCES. Economics Information Guide Series, vol. 7. Detroit: Gale Research Co., 1977.

Annotated bibliography of journal articles. Covers public health, disease, and illness-specific analyses.

1.44 Andrews, Theodora. A BIBLIOGRAPHY OF THE SOCIOECONOMIC ASPECTS OF MEDICINE. Littleton, Colo.: Libraries Unlimited, 1975.

General References

Includes materials that have social, political, and economic implications. Limited to English-language materials. Includes reference books and monographs, a few pamphlets, annuals, and statistical services.

1.45 Culyer, A.J., et al. AN ANNOTATED BIBLIOGRAPHY OF HEALTH ECONOMICS: ENGLISH LANGUAGE SOURCES. New York: St. Martin's Press, 1977.

References to some journal articles and government publications which include statistical information. Includes supply of health services, estimating the cost of disease, and measuring the output of health services.

1.46 Frank, Nathalie D. "After Statistical Abstract--What?" RQ 14 (Spring 1975): 204-10.

Discussion of guides to federal statistical publications. Includes guides to specialized abstracts, subject indexes, and data files. Includes list of sixty-four references.

1.47 Jensen, Marilyn Anne. "Selected Sources of Current Population, Vital, and Health Statistics." BULLETIN OF THE MEDICAL LIBRARY ASSOCIATION 60 (January 1972): 14-21.

Covers local and state publications for California as well as major federal and international publications.

1.48 Lufburrow, Nancy C. "Social Indicators; Or Selected Federal Social Statistical Programs." RQ 16 (Summer 1977): 301-6.

Describes some of the newer federal health and other statistical series. Excellent bibliography of fifty-six references.

1.49 Sax, Ellen. DISTRIBUTION OF HEALTH PERSONNEL: AN ANNOTATED BIBLIOGRAPHY. New York: National Health Council, 1976.

Cites publications pertaining to the distribution of health personnel, factors influencing location of practitioners, and incentive programs to practice in underserved areas. A state-by-state listing in section 1 and a subject listing in section 2.

1.50 SELECTED NATIONAL DATA SOURCES FOR HEALTH PLANNERS. DHEW publication no. (HRA) 76-1236. Washington, D.C.: Government Printing Office, 1976.

Updates and expands an earlier sourcebook, SELECTED DATA SETS FOR HEALTH PLANNERS, volume I. Provides publishing agency, data and periodicity, geographic areas covered, population covered, and data elements for each data source. Includes both publications and data tapes. Covers health statis-

General References

tics, health status, manpower, facilities, services, health economics, and demographic data.

1.51 Silberg, Nancy. DATA FOR HEALTH PLANNING: A SELECTED ANNOTATED BIBLIOGRAPHY. Monticello, Ill.: Council of Planning Librarians, 1974.

A selected bibliography of books, pamphlets, and articles which contain data useful for health planning. Includes one section on sources of data and another section which lists sources of data by subject such as demographic, health services, and vital statistics.

1.52 U.S. Bureau of Health Manpower. AN ANNOTATED BIBLIOGRAPHY OF PUBLICATIONS. Hyattsville, Md.: 1977.

"The publications listed relate largely to health manpower supply and requirements and are designed to contribute to a better understanding of health manpower issues, developments, trends and projections." Gives availability and price for each item.

1.53 U.S. Bureau of Health Manpower. Division of Nursing. INTERAGENCY CONFERENCE ON NURSING STATISTICS: ABSTRACTS OF STUDIES. DHEW publication no. (HRA) 75-24. Washington, D.C.: Government Printing Office, 1975.

Abstracts of studies relating to nursing manpower. Contains data on nurses, nursing education, and the system within which nurses practice. Lists basic nursing statistics sourcebooks.

1.54 U.S. Bureau of Health Planning and Resources Development. GUIDE TO DATA FOR HEALTH SYSTEMS PLANNERS. Health Planning Information Series, vol. 2. HRP-0007376. Springfield, Va.: National Technical Information Service, 1976.

Prepared by the Census Bureau to assist local health system agencies. Presents descriptions and bibliographic information of major statistical series on population trends, vital statistics, morbidity and disability indexes, inpatient facilities, ambulatory care, and home care.

1.55 U.S. Bureau of Labor Statistics. DIRECTORY OF DATA SOURCES ON RACIAL AND ETHNIC MINORITIES. BLS Bulletin 1879. Washington, D.C.: Government Printing Office, 1975.

Provides users of statistics on racial and ethnic minority groups with annotated references to sources of data published by the federal government. Includes data sources such as publications presenting social and economic characteristics of minority groups

General References

for the nation and selected areas based primarily on household surveys. Does not cover vital and health statistics and arrest and prison population statistics. Divided into four major sections: blacks, persons of Spanish ancestry, other races, and other ethnic groups.

1.56 U.S. Bureau of the Census. DIRECTORY OF FEDERAL STATISTICS FOR LOCAL AREAS: A GUIDE TO SOURCES. Washington, D.C.: Government Printing Office, 1978.

Presents information in chart form by subject, tabular detail, geographic areas, frequency, and publication source. Designed to show users where to find data on small geographic areas (counties, cities, and neighborhoods). Includes publications for period 1966-76. Appendixes on the availability of unpublished statistics on microfilm, data files, and special tabulations. Includes annotated list of seventy-five guides to federal and municipal data.

1.57 U.S. National Center for Health Statistics. FACTS AT YOUR FINGERTIPS: A GUIDE TO SOURCES OF STATISTICAL INFORMATION ON MAJOR HEALTH TOPICS. Hyattsville, Md.: 1977-- . Annual.

Lists major sources of statistical information on major health topics including vital statistics, chronic diseases, manpower, and utilization. Under each topic, cites the NCHS publications first, followed by other HEW sources, other federal agencies, and by private organizations or associations.

1.58 U.S. National Clearinghouse on Alcohol Information. SELECTED PUBLICATIONS ON STATISTICS AND DEMOGRAPHIC RESEARCH ON ALCOHOL USE AND ABUSE: INCLUDING STATISTICS AND DEMOGRAPHY. ADM 76-272. Washington, D.C.: 1976.

Annotated bibliography of demographic studies of alcohol use and abuse.

1.58a U.S. National Library of Medicine. NATIONAL LIBRARY OF MEDICINE CURRENT CATALOG. Washington, D.C.: Government Printing Office, 1966-- . Quarterly.

A computer produced catalog of publications catalogued at the National Library of Medicine, regardless of date of imprint, except pre-1801 and Americana titles. Main subject and author sections for both monographs and serials. Annual and quinquennial cumulations.

1.59 Weise, Frieda [O.]. A BIBLIOGRAPHIC GUIDE TO STATISTICS AND HEALTH PLANNING INFORMATION. PB 269-718. Springfield, Va.: National Technical Information Service, 1977.

General References

Selected annotated bibliography meant to be a guide for librarians, students, and health planners. Geared toward Illinois with state and local documents cited, although not to the exclusion of federal documents and private agencies and publishers. Periodical citations excluded.

INDEXES AND ABSTRACTING SERVICES

This section presents publications providing access to current literature on specific topics of health statistics. The major indexing and abstracting services which contain references to journal articles, government publications or other types of publications are included.

The most comprehensive source for U.S. statistical publications is the AMERICAN STATISTICS INDEX/ABSTRACT (see no. 1.61). It provides extremely detailed access to all statistical publications of the federal government. The CURRENT LISTING AND TOPICAL INDEX TO THE VITAL AND HEALTH STATISTICS SERIES (see no. 1.71) is also quite useful as is FACTS AT YOUR FINGERTIPS (see no. 1.57). Especially good for access to journal literature are the HOSPITAL LITERATURE INDEX (see no. 1.66) and MEDSOC (see no. 1.68).

It should be remembered that journal articles will usually not provide comprehensive statistics. These are generally the published results of surveys, sampling studies, or experiments which are limited to small populations. However, for some subjects, especially chronic diseases and cost data, they contribute the best information available.

1.60 ABSTRACTS OF HEALTH CARE MANAGEMENT STUDIES. Cooperative Information Center for Hospital Management Studies, University of Michigan, School of Public Health, Ann Arbor, Mich. 48104, vol. 15, 1978-- . Quarterly.

> Formerly: ABSTRACTS OF HOSPITAL MANAGEMENT STUDIES. Abstracts studies not likely to be in other indexes. Some unpublished works and studies made under auspices of university, government, or hospital research institutions. Includes statistical studies. Subject categories of interest are: chronic disease facilities and programs, health services, utilization and need, supply and cost, manpower resources and utilization. Studies available on microfilm or as photocopies through University Microfilms International.

1.61 AMERICAN STATISTICS INDEX: A COMPREHENSIVE GUIDE AND INDEX TO THE STATISTICAL PUBLICATIONS OF THE U.S. GOVERNMENT. Congressional Information Service, 7101 Wisconsin Avenue, N.W., Washington, D.C. 20014, 1974-- . Monthly.

> A major index to American statistics. Intended to identify all statistical data published by the federal government, to

General References

catalog publications in which data appear, to describe the contents fully, to index in full subject detail, and to micropublish the publications indexed. Includes subject, author, title, agency report numbers indexes. Also indexed by categories: geographic, economic, and demographic. Published in two parts both monthly and annually: indexes and abstracts. Available online commercially.

1.62 BIBLIOGRAPHY ON HEALTH INDEXES. Clearinghouse on Health Indexes. National Center for Health Statistics, 3700 East-West Highway, Hyattsville, Md., 1974-- . Quarterly.

Established to provide information which will be helpful in developing composite health measures. Accordingly, the following definition of health index has been adopted: "a health index is a measure which purports to reflect the health status of an individual or defined groups." Includes a selection of documents in the clearinghouse file such as journal articles, books, conference proceedings, government publications, and reports on grants and contracts.

1.63 EXCERPTA MEDICA, SECTION 17: PUBLIC HEALTH, SOCIAL MEDICINE, AND HYGIENE. Excerpta Medica, Keizersgracht 305, Box 1126, Amsterdam, Holland, 1975-- . 20 times yearly.

Abstracts current international journal literature. Devotes chapter 2 of this abstract to statistics including demography, morbidity, mortality, and vital statistics. Other subjects of interest: industrial medicine, accidents, occupational diseases, and poisoning. Detailed subject index. Uses the term statistics both as a subheading and major subject heading. Annual cumulated index. Available online commercially.

1.64 EXCERPTA MEDICA, SECTION 36: HEALTH ECONOMICS AND HOSPITAL MANAGEMENT. Excerpta Medica, Keizersgracht 305, Box 1126, Amsterdam, Holland, 1971-- . 20 times yearly.

Abstracts current international journal literature. Very detailed subject index leads to statistical articles. Uses term statistics both as a subheading and a major subject heading. Annual cumulated index. Available online commercially.

1.65 HEALTH PLANNING: WEEKLY GOVERNMENT ABSTRACT. National Technical Information Service, 5285 Port Royal Road, Springfield, Va. 22161, 1975-- .

Abstract prepared in collaboration with the National Health Planning Information Center (NHPIC) in the Bureau of Health Planning and Resources Development, Health Resources Administration. Includes documents relating to health services and

General References

health needs; health services and facilities utilization; health manpower requirements, utilization, and education; health related costs; methods of health services funding; and government and private agency activities relating to health planning and resources development. Publications available in both microfiche and hard copy from NTIS. Available online commercially. Final issue annual subject index.

1.66 HOSPITAL LITERATURE INDEX. American Hospital Association, 840 North Lake Shore Drive, Chicago, Ill. 60611, 1945-- . Quarterly.

Citations in this index cover the delivery of health care in all types of health care facilities. Also covers economics, planning, health insurance, manpower, services, and utilization. Since March 1978, subject headings according to National Library of Medicine's Medical Subject Headings (MESH). HEALTH PLANNING AND ADMINISTRATION, the online version of this index.

1.67 INDEX MEDICUS. National Library of Medicine, 8600 Rockville Pike, Bethesda, Md. 20014 (Available from: Superintendent of Documents, Government Printing Office, Washington, D.C. 20402), 1960-- . Monthly

Currently indexes 3,000 of the world's foremost biomedical journals as well as selected monographs. Subjects indexed primarily clinical in nature. Statistical articles also listed under the relevant main heading with one of the following subheadings: occurrence, supply and distribution, mortality, manpower, or utilization. Annual cumulation. MEDLINE, the online data base.

1.68 MEDICAL SOCIOECONOMIC RESEARCH SOURCES (MEDSOC). American Medical Association, 535 North Dearborn, Chicago, Ill. 60610, 1963-- . Quarterly.

Formerly: INDEX TO THE LITERATURE OF MEDICAL SOCIO-ECONOMICS. A guide to the publications in the sociology and economics of medicine. Covers all types of publications including journals, newspapers, books, pamphlets, and government publications. Subject headings of interest for statistical sources: morbidity, mortality, vital statistics, health care services, utilization, economics, medical care, health manpower, and statistics.

1.69 MEDOC: A COMPUTERIZED INDEX TO U.S. GOVERNMENT DOCUMENTS IN THE MEDICAL AND HEALTH SCIENCES. Eccles Medical Sciences Library, Salt Lake City, Utah 84112, vol. 1, 1968-71; vol. 2, 1975-- . Quarterly.

General References

Covers a selection of relevant documents giving Superintendent of Documents number, title, subject, series, and agency. Tells whether it is a pamphlet, and gives price. Includes statistics as subject heading. Does not include technical reports. Eccles is a depository library. Available online commercially.

1.70   POPULATION INDEX. Office of Population Research, Woodrow Wilson School of Public and International Affairs, Princeton University, Princeton, N.J. 08540, 1935-- . Quarterly.

Covers international demographic research; includes a geographic index. Subject headings: general population studies and theory, trends in population size, spatial distribution, fertility, demographic and economic interpretations, mortality, and vital rates. Also lists official statistical publications of foreign countries, the United States, individual states, and bibliographies.

1.71   U.S. National Center for Health Statistics. CURRENT LISTING AND TOPICAL INDEX TO THE VITAL AND HEALTH STATISTICS SERIES, 1962-78. DHEW publication no. (PHS) 79-1301, Hyattsville, Md.: 1979.

An index to health topics covered in the VITAL AND HEALTH STATISTICS SERIES and an index to the presentation of data according to demographic and socioeconomic variables. Organized in two sections, with some overlapping. Topics and variables related to the health status of people in section 1. Characteristics of health facilities and manpower in section 2. Includes list of titles appearing in the VITAL AND HEALTH STATISTICS SERIES (see no. 1.89) and VITAL STATISTICS ADVANCE DATA (see no. 2.13). Updated periodically.

1.72   Zeisset, Paul T. INDEX TO SELECTED 1970 CENSUS REPORTS. Washington, D.C.: U.S. Bureau of the Census, 1974.

Reference guide designed to facilitate use of the reports from the 1970 Censuses of Population and Housing and to increase understanding of the scope of the census tabulations available in print.

MACHINE-READABLE FILES

Machine-readable data files should be distinguished from machine readable bibliographic files. The former contain raw or primary data generally not available in printed form, while the latter contain only bibliographic information.

This section is divided into three subsections. The first presents guides to both types of files available from the public and from the private sector. The second part lists two examples of data files commercially available. The third lists

General References

bibliographic files also available commercially. Among the guides, the most comprehensive list of bibliographic files is the DIRECTORY OF ONLINE INFORMATION RESOURCES (see no. 1.73), while the most complete listing of government data files is the DIRECTORY OF COMPUTERIZED DATA FILES (see no. 1.80).

Guides to Machine-Readable Files

1.73 Capital Systems Group. DIRECTORY OF ONLINE INFORMATION RESOURCES. Rockville, Md.: 1978. 1977-- . Semiannual.

Describes data bases commercially available. Includes data bases that provide primary information as well as those that provide bibliographic information.

1.74 U.S. Bureau of Health Manpower. AREA RESOURCE FILE: A MANPOWER PLANNING AND RESEARCH TOOL. DHEW publication no. (HRA) 77-23. Hyattsville, Md.: 1977.

User guide that describes the content and format of the area resources file, a computerized system providing demographic, health status, and health resources data for each county and SMSA. Includes national summary, basic area profiles, and manpower-population ratio. Appendixes of all data inputs.

1.75 U.S. Bureau of Labor Statistics. BLS DATA BANK FILES AND STATISTICAL ROUTINES. Report 507. Washington, D.C.: Government Printing Office, 1978.

Contains data file descriptions which summarize published data stored in each file of the BLS Data Bank.

1.76 U.S. Bureau of the Census. INDEX TO 1970 CENSUS SUMMARY TAPES. By Paul T. Zeisset. Washington, D.C.: Government Printing Office, 1973.

An index with cross reference guides to all tabulations in all six "counts" of the 1970 census summary data, organized alphabetically by subject variable.

1.77 _____. SUMMARY TAPE PROCESSING CENTERS. Washington, D.C.: 1978.

An address list of organizations who have obtained 1970 census tapes. Lists centers that perform processing services for data users. Since the centers are not supported by the Census Bureau, fees and services vary. Listed alphabetically by state.

General References

1.78   U.S. National Center for Health Services Research. HEALTH SERVICES R & D DATA TAPES. DHEW publication no. (HRA) 76-3155. Rockville, Md.: 1977.

   Brochure describing eight data tapes and giving availability and price. Data from studies done over the past eight years on utilization of health services and health care costs.

1.79   U.S. National Center for Health Statistics. STANDARDIZED MICRO-DATA TAPE TRANSCRIPTS. DHEW publication no. (PHS) 78-1213. Washington, D.C.: Government Printing Office, 1978.

   Describes microdata tapes available for purchase from the National Center for Health Statistics. Lists tapes meant to fill the need of consumers who require data in a format or detail not provided in the center's publications. Describes, in detail, the content of each data set. Gives purchase price that includes costs of the magnetic tape volumes, the printed materials explaining tape content, and the documentation necessary to utilize the files.

1.80   U.S. National Technical Information Service. A DIRECTORY OF COMPUTERIZED DATA FILES, SOFTWARE, AND RELATED TECHNICAL REPORTS. NTIS/SR-78/03. Springfield, Va.: 1978.

   Guide to machine-readable data files, data bases and software available to the public from federal agencies. Also includes printed reports of pertinent data. Covers demography and population, health care, health statistics, and social services. Gives availability, price, and item type.

Data Files

1.80a   HAS-MONITREND

   Data for hospital management collected by the American Hospital Association (AHA), Hospital Administrative Services (HAS) on a monthly basis for a fee from participating institutions. Currently serves 2,800 hospitals, 400 nursing homes, and 50 ambulatory care centers. Includes data on costs and expenditures, staffing, revenue, patient days, and many other items useful to management. Sends reports of monthly indicators to participating institutions. Summarized data in the SIX-MONTH NATIONAL DATA BOOK available by subscription from the AHA.

1.80b   PAS-MAP

   Professional Activity Study-Medial Audit Program (PAS-MAP), a computerized information system provided by the Commission on Professional and Hospital Activities (CPHA). Nationally

General References

available to support medical care evaluation studies by providing access to information in medical records. Collects routine data from patient records such as: (1) results of admission investigations; (2) whether laboratory tests, x-rays, and other diagnostic tests were performed; (3) categories of drugs administered; and (4) whether other therapeutic services were provided. Presently serves more than 2,200 hospitals in the United States. Prepares monthly and annual reports for participating institutions.

Bibliographic Files

Machine-readable bibliographic files provide rapid access to current references from the literature. They also provide the ability to manipulate subjects in a variety of combinations leading to references which would be difficult to retrieve from a printed index or bibliography. Of the files listed here, the two most useful in obtaining references to publications containing health statistics are ASI (see no. 1.81) and HEALTH (see no. 1.84). As noted before, ASI provides citations and abstracts to all federal statistical publications—a major source in the field. HEALTH, available only since 1 November 1978, is extremely pertinent with its emphasis on health planning literature.

The annotations here are relatively short since the printed version of each data base was described in the previous section, "Indexes and Abstracting Services." Appendix E lists the names and addresses of suppliers from whom these bibliographic files are available.

1.81   ASI.

Covers statistical publications of the U.S. government comprehensively. Prepared by the Congressional Information Service. Corresponds to the AMERICAN STATISTICS INDEX (see no. 1.61). Covers 1973 to the present. Citation and abstract in Unit Record. Supplier is SDC (Systems Development Corporation).

1.82   CATLINE.

Contains references to books and serials cataloged at the National Library of Medicine and is part of the Medical Literature Analysis and Retrieval System (MEDLARS). Printed version CURRENT CATALOG (see no. 1.58A). Covers 1965 to the present. Citation with full cataloging information and NLM call number in Unit Record. Supplier is the National Library of Medicine.

General References

1.83 EXCERPTA MEDICA.

Covers worldwide research literature in the health sciences. Prepared by the Excerpta Medica Foundation. Corresponds to the printed EXCERPTA MEDICA (see nos. 1.63-64). Covers 1975 to the present. Unit Record has citation and abstract. Supplier is Lockheed.

1.84 HEALTH.

Full title HEALTH PLANNING AND ADMINISTRATION. Citations covering all aspects of health care delivery are from journals indexed for MEDLINE (see no. 1.85), HOSPITAL LITERATURE INDEX (see no. 1.66), and other journals selected for their emphasis on health care matters. Will eventually include references to nonserial items such as technical reports from the National Health Planning Information Center. Part of MEDLARS. Produced by the National Library of Medicine in cooperation with the American Hospital Association and the Health Resources Administration. Covers 1975 to the present. Citation and abstract in Unit Record. Supplier is the National Library of Medicine.

1.85 MEDLINE.

Covers biomedical journal articles from 3,000 journals published in the United States and seventy foreign countries. Includes a limited number of chapters from selected monographs. Prepared by the National Library of Medicine. Used to publish INDEX MEDICUS (see 1.67). Covers current and two preceding years. Backfiles to 1966. Citation and English abstract in Unit Record, if published with the article. Suppliers are the National Library of Medicine and Bibliographic Retrieval Services.

1.86 MEDOC.

Provides access to U.S. government publications in medicine and health related fields including many statistical publications. Produced by the Eccles Health Sciences Library at the University of Utah which is a depository library. Corresponds to the printed MEDOC (see no. 1.69). Covers 1968 to the present. Citation, including Superintendent of Documents number, in Unit Record. Supplier is Bibliographic Retrieval Services.

1.87 NTIS.

Contains citations to U.S. government-sponsored research and development technical reports. Produced by the National Technical Information Service. Corresponds to HEALTH PLANNING: WEEKLY GOVERNMENT ABSTRACTS (see no. 1.65) and the biweekly GOVERNMENT REPORTS ANNOUNCEMENTS.

General References

Covers 1970 to the present. Citation and abstract in Unit Record. Suppliers are Bibliographic Retrieval Services, Lockheed, and SDC (Systems Development Corporation).

COMPILATIONS OF HEALTH STATISTICS

The publications in this section are compilations of health statistics. They include government publications, and publications of private organizations and private publishers, showing the diverse sources of health statistics.

Vital and Health Statistics Series

This subsection presents collections of vital and health statistics series from 1936 to the present in order to provide a historical continuum for this information. The U.S. Bureau of the Census was originally charged with the task of collecting vital statistics; however, this is now the responsibility of the National Center for Health Statistics. The subjects of the collections and publication series have expanded over the years to cover not only vital statistics, but morbidity, health resources, utilization of health resources, and family growth as well.

1.88   U.S. Bureau of the Census. VITAL STATISTICS--SPECIAL REPORTS. Vols. 1-54. Washington, D.C.: 1936-65.

Superseded by the National Health Survey Series, A-D (below). Covers all aspects of vital statistics with trend analyses over a period of years, special data on unusual causes of death, and demographic studies.

1.89   U.S. National Center for Health Statistics. VITAL AND HEALTH STATISTICS SERIES. Washington, D.C.: Government Printing Office, 1963-- . Irregular.

Data covered by the surveys and studies of the National Center for Health Statistics compiled and published in a number of series. Sometimes called the "Rainbow Series." Series 1-4 supersedes HEALTH STATISTICS SERIES A and D of the National Health Survey and Series 10-12 replace HEALTH STATISTICS SERIES B and C of the National Health Survey. The "Rainbow Series" are listed below.

Series 1: PROGRAM AND COLLECTION PROCEDURES, 1963-- . Reports which describe the general programs of the National Center for Health Statistics.

Series 2: DATA EVALUATION AND METHODS RESEARCH, 1963-- . Studies of new statistical methodology including: experimental tests of new survey methods, and studies of vital statistics collection methods.

General References

Series 3: ANALYTICAL STUDIES, 1964-- . Reports presenting analytical or interpretive studies based on vital and health statistics.

Series 4: DOCUMENTS AND COMMITTEE REPORTS, 1965-- . Final reports of major committees concerned with vital and health statistics.

Series 10: DATA FROM THE HEALTH INTERVIEW SURVEY, 1963--. Statistics on illness, accidental injuries, disability, use of hospitals, medical, dental, and other services, based on data collected in national household interview survey.

Series 11: DATA FROM THE HEALTH EXAMINATION SURVEY AND THE HEALTH AND NUTRITION EXAMINATION SURVEY, 1964-- .

Series 12: DATA FROM THE HEALTH RECORDS SURVEY, no. 1-24, 1965-74. Reports on the health characteristics of persons in institutions, and on hospital, medical nursing, and personal care received. Discontinued. Reports absorbed into series 13.

Series 13: DATA ON HEALTH RESOURCES UTILIZATION, 1966-- . Statistics relating to discharged patients in short-stay hospitals, based on a sample of patient records in a national sample of hospitals.

Series 14: DATA ON HEALTH RESOURCES: MANPOWER AND FACILITIES, 1968-- . Statistics on the numbers, geographic distribution, and characteristics of health resources including physicians, dentists, nurses, other health manpower occupations, hospitals, nursing homes, and outpatient and other inpatient facilities.

Series 20: DATA ON MORTALITY, 1965-- . Various special reports on mortality giving data on other than that in the annual volume of VITAL STATISTICS REPORTS. Covers tabulations by cause of death, age, and data for geographic areas.

Series 21: DATA ON NATALITY, MARRIAGE AND DIVORCE, 1965-- . Data on birth by age of mother, birth order, geographic areas, states, cities, and time series of rates.

Series 22: DATA FROM THE NATIONAL NATALITY AND MORTALITY SURVEYS, no. 1-15, 1961-76. Discontinued. Reports absorbed into series 20 and 21.

Series 23: DATA FROM THE NATIONAL SURVEY OF FAMILY GROWTH, 1977-- . Data on fertility, family planning, and those aspects of maternal and child health related to childbearing.

1.90 U.S. National Health Survey. HEALTH STATISTICS SERIES A. No. 1-4. Public Health Service publication no. 584-A. Washington, D.C.: 1958-62.

Program descriptions, survey designs, concepts, and definitions.

General References

1.91 _____. HEALTH STATISTICS SERIES B. No. 1-42. Public Health Service publication no. 584-B. Washington, D.C.: 1958-63.

    Health interview survey results by topic.

1.92 _____. HEALTH STATISTICS SERIES C. No. 1-7. Public Health Service publication no. 584-C. Washington, D.C.: 1959-62.

    Health interview surveys for different population groups.

1.93 _____. HEALTH STATISTICS SERIES D. No. 1-8. Public Health Service publication no. 584-D. Washington, D.C.: 1960-63.

    Evaluation reports concerning the program.

GENERAL COMPILATIONS

The publications in this subsection cover all topics of health statistics. Particularly useful compilations are HEALTH: UNITED STATES (see no. 1.110), MEDICAL RISKS (see no. 1.100), and the STANDARD MEDICAL ALMANAC (see no. 1.101) since they provide data as well as information concerning the sources of data. Not to be overlooked for data on chronic diseases is THE KILLERS AND CRIPPLERS (see no. 1.98).

Although the main thrust of this bibliography is United States data, several publications covering foreign countries have been included. Especially noteworthy are the EUROHEALTH HANDBOOK (see no. 1.97) and the SYNCRISIS Series (see no. 1.115).

1.94 American Medical Association. REFERENCE DATA ON THE PROFILE OF MEDICAL PRACTICE. Chicago: 1971-- . Annual.

    Contains papers prepared by the staff on issues of current importance to the practice of medicine and data on physician manpower, utilization of services and physicians' income, expenses, and fees. Gives sources.

1.95 American Public Health Association. MINORITY HEALTH CHART BOOK. Washington, D.C.: Government Printing Office, 1975.

    Gives a graphic overview of and highlights key facts about several major racial and ethnic minorities in the United States, particularly health status and needs, utilization of health services, and involvement in health resources. Shows differences in data between these minorities and the white population.

1.96 Axelrod, S.J.; Donabedian, A.; and Gentry, D.W. MEDICAL CARE CHART BOOK. 6th ed. Ann Arbor: University of Michigan, 1976.

    Covers a large range of data topics. Presents data on a national level from sources noted in the book. Covers popu-

General References

lation characteristics, mortality and morbidity, receipt of care, costs and expenditures, health personnel, facilities, quality of care, tax-supported medical care programs, and medical care insurance.

1.97 EUROHEALTH HANDBOOK. New York: Robert S. First, 1971-- . Annual.

Health data for West European countries including health care expenditures, hospital statistics, health personnel, and morbidity and mortality. Lists source publications and publishers as well as government health agencies and addresses.

1.98 National Health Education Committee. THE KILLERS AND CRIPPLERS: FACTS ON MAJOR DISEASES IN THE U.S. TODAY. 11th ed. New York: McKay, 1976.

A sourcebook of statistics on the principal causes of death and disability in the United States. Presents data to evaluate progress against these diseases and points out areas where more funds for research are needed. Covers allergies and infectious diseases, arthritis and rheumatism, blinding eye diseases, cancer, cerebral palsy, deafness, digestive diseases, epilepsy, genetic disease, hypertension, mental illness and retardation, multiple sclerosis, muscular dystrophy, Parkinsonism, disability, and tuberculosis.

1.99 REFERENCE DATA ON SOCIOECONOMIC ISSUES OF HEALTH. Chicago: 1971-- . Annual.

Presents tables and charts on general health services topics. Gives data on characteristics of the U.S. population (age, sex, and race), morbidity, and mortality, characteristics of the health services delivery system, and financing mechanisms.

1.99A Rowland, Howard S. THE NURSES ALMANAC. Germantown, Md.: Aspen Systems Corporation, 1978.

A comprehensive handbook of facts about and for nurses. Includes statistics on the cost of health care, nursing manpower, nursing education, hospitals, nursing homes, diseases, the aged, the handicapped, women, and minorities.

1.100 Singer, Richard B., and Levenson, Louis, eds. MEDICAL RISKS: PATTERNS OF MORTALITY AND SURVIVAL. Lexington, Mass.: Heath, 1976.

Compilation of mortality and survival statistics in relation to risk factors identified in groups of people in follow-up observation. Lists causes of death with a description and a list of studies containing mortality and survival statistics for the cause

General References

in part 1. Abstracts of studies listed in part 1 with tables of statistics in part 2.

1.101 STANDARD MEDICAL ALMANAC. Chicago: Marquis Academic Media, 1977.

Provides a comprehensive picture of the health care industry in the United States. Contains narrative as well as statistical data concerning health manpower, income and expenditures, education and licensure, facilities, disease, and the federal government and health.

1.102 STATISTICAL ABSTRACT OF THE UNITED STATES. Washington, D.C.: Government Printing Office, 1889-- . Annual.

Annual standard summary of statistics on the social, political, and economic organization of the United States designed to serve as a convenient volume for statistical reference and as a guide to other statistical publications and sources. Major sections of interest include population, vital statistics, education, income, and labor force.

1.103 SURGERY IN THE UNITED STATES: A SUMMARY REPORT ON SURGICAL SERVICES FOR THE UNITED STATES. 3 vols. Chicago: The American College of Surgeons and the American Surgical Association, 1976.

Comprehensive report covering surgical manpower; utilization of surgical procedures; and organization, delivery, and financing of surgical services. Majority of each volume consists of statistical information in the form of charts, graphs, and tables.

1.104 United Nations. Statistical Office. DEMOGRAPHIC YEARBOOK. New York: 1949-- . Annual.

Offers official demographic statistics from 250 geographic entities of the world. Different field of demographic statistics receives intensive treatment each year. Includes tables on population, natality, fetal and infant mortality, general mortality, life tables, nuptiality, divorce, and international migration.

1.105 _____. STATISTICAL YEARBOOK. New York: 1949-- . Annual.

Compilation of international statistics. Includes tables on population, economic activity, manpower, agriculture, forestry, fishing, industrial production, mining, manufacturing, energy construction, transport, communications, consumption, finance, and culture. Statistics arranged by country and by continent.

1.106 U.S. Bureau of the Census. HISTORICAL STATISTICS OF THE UNITED STATES: COLONIAL TIMES TO 1970. Washington, D.C.: Government Printing Office, 1976.

General References

Brings together historical series of wide general interest and informs the user where additional data can be found. Supplements the annual STATISTICAL ABSTRACT OF THE UNITED STATES (see no. 1.102). Excellent chapters on "Population," and "Vital Statistics and Health and Medical Care" with sources of statistics given.

1.107 U.S. Congress. Congressional Budget Office. HEALTH DIFFERENTIALS BETWEEN WHITE AND NONWHITE AMERICANS. Washington, D.C.: Government Printing Office, 1977.

Data for this study were drawn from various sources including unpublished data from NCHS Health Interview Survey. Tables present data on selected measures of health status, trends in health status, and utilization of health services, all by race.

1.108 U.S. Congress. House of Representatives. Committee on Ways and Means. NATIONAL HEALTH INSURANCE RESOURCE BOOK. Rev. ed. Washington, D.C.: Government Printing Office, 1976.

Extensive collection of statistics concerning the health care field. Includes information on health services and facilities, health manpower, health insurance, patients, and delivery systems of other nations.

1.109 U.S. Department of Commerce. SOCIAL INDICATORS, 1976. Washington, D.C.: Government Printing Office, 1977.

Collection of statistics describes social conditions and trends in the United States. Examines life expectancy, disability, and access to medical care. Also covers public safety, education, employment, income, housing, leisure and recreation, and population.

1.110 U.S. Health Resources Administration. HEALTH: UNITED STATES. Washington, D.C.: Government Printing Office, 1975-76-- . Annual.

Annual report by the secretary of the Department of Health, Education, and Welfare to the president and the Congress as required by the Public Health Service Act. Includes analytical chapters on specific health topics as well as many statistical tables on the nation's health with expository text. Gives data sources and a glossary.

1.111 _____. HEALTH OF THE DISADVANTAGED: A CHARTBOOK. DHEW publication no. (HRA) 77-628. Washington, D.C.: Government Printing Office, 1977.

Chartbook on racial minorities' health status, health services utilization, health manpower, and health care financing. Data for 1970-75. Charts and tables show data by race, income,

General References

education, sex, age, region, SMSA and non-SMSA, and poverty status.

1.112 U.S. National Center for Health Statistics. HEALTH IN THE LATER YEARS OF LIFE--SELECTED DATA FROM THE NATIONAL CENTER FOR HEALTH STATISTICS. Washington, D.C.: Government Printing Office, 1971.

Includes charts on three areas. First, life and death tables such as mortality and life expectancy, major causes of death, and divorce rates. Second, health problems such as chronic conditions, acute conditions, activity limitation, and disability. Third, utilization of health services such as physician and dentist visits, hospital and nursing home care, and care at home.

1.113 U.S. National Clearinghouse on Aging. STATISTICAL REPORTS ON OLDER AMERICANS. Rockville, Md.: 1977-- . Irregular.

Series of reports on the socioeconomic conditions of the elderly, including income levels, employment, living arrangements, health care, and population trends. Data from census reports and other publications.

1.114 U.S. National Institute on Aging. EPIDEMIOLOGY OF AGING. DHEW publication no. (NIH) 75-711. Washington, D.C.: Government Printing Office, 1975.

Compilation of papers on medical aspects of aging, including life expectancy, mortality rates, causes of death, and demographic and socioeconomic characteristics of the population over sixty-five.

1.115 U.S. Public Health Service. Office of International Health. SYNCRISIS: THE DYNAMICS OF HEALTH, AN ANALYTIC SERIES ON THE INTERACTIONS OF HEALTH AND SOCIOECONOMIC DEVELOPMENT. Washington, D.C.: 1970-- . Irregular.

Reports cover developing nations and stress the relationship between health and socioeconomic development. All contain data on: population size and trends, mortality and morbidity, costs of disease, nutritional problems, and health resources. Includes twenty-four countries in individual volumes thus far.

1.116 World Health Organization. WORLD HEALTH STATISTICS ANNUAL. 3 vols. 1965-- . Annual.

Supersedes the ANNUAL EPIDEMIOLOGICAL AND VITAL STATISTICS SERIES. Published in three separate volumes: Volume 1, VITAL STATISTICS AND CAUSES OF DEATH;

General References

volume 2, INFECTIOUS DISEASES: CASES, DEATHS AND VACCINATIONS; and volume 3, HEALTH PERSONNEL AND HOSPITAL ESTABLISHMENTS. Gives information on the population and general vital statistics of countries and territories in volume 1. Gives numbers of deaths and death rates by age, cause, and sex. Gives information on infectious diseases, including cases, deaths, and number of vaccinations in volume 2. Also seasonal variations for some diseases and the sex and age distribution. Contains statistics on health personnel and hospital establishments including the number of personnel working in each country in volume 3. Shows numbers of physicians in various specialties for each country as well as paramedical personnel. Also presents numbers of types of hospitals as well as numbers of beds for each type.

1.117 _____. WORLD HEALTH STATISTICS REPORT. Geneva: 1947-- . Quarterly.

Report supplements the WORLD HEALTH STATISTICS ANNUAL (see no. 1.116) and contains two parts: Part 1, "Special Subjects," contains detailed analyses of subjects of current interest in the areas of vital or health and health-related topics. Part 2, "Current Data," gives recent statistics on infectious diseases, vital statistics, health personnel, hospital establishments, and health expenditures.

Chapter 2
VITAL STATISTICS

This chapter presents the official vital statistics publications of the U.S. National Center for Health Statistics as well as its predecessor, the U.S. Bureau of the Census. Publications of other federal agencies pertaining to vital statistics have also been included.

Vital statistics, including births, deaths, marriages, and divorces, are compiled for the country as a whole by the U.S. National Center for Health Statistics. Reports of births and deaths originate with the attending physician (or other health care attendant). These are sent to the local health department which in turn sends them on to the state department for its information and recording. The state health department sends duplicate reports to the federal health authority, the U.S. National Center for Health Statistics, Public Health Service, and U.S. Department of Health, Education, and Welfare. Marriage and divorce information also originates with the local agency, usually the county, and is sent to the state health department which in turn sends it to the U.S. Public Health Service.

Although each state has a law requiring registration of births, deaths, and fetal deaths, these laws are not uniformly observed. Annual collection of mortality statistics began in 1900 with the establishment of registration areas. (Before that, they were collected during the decennial census.) But not all states were admitted until 1933 due to the lack of uniformity. Natality registration areas began in 1915 and included all states by 1933. To date, only forty-seven states and the District of Columbia are included in the marriage registration area and only twenty-nine states in the divorce registration areas. The varying coverage in the past has made it difficult to obtain reliable data.

The definitive and final tabulations of vital statistics appear in the annual volumes, VITAL STATISTICS OF THE UNITED STATES (see no. 2.14). However, there is a time lag of about four years in their publication. Provisional and current figures appear in the MONTHLY VITAL STATISTICS (see no. 2.10) and MORBIDITY AND MORTALITY WEEKLY REPORT (see no. 2.6).

Vital Statistics

2.1   Grove, Robert D., and Hetzel, Alice M. VITAL STATISTICS RATES IN THE UNITED STATES, 1940-60. PHS publication no. 1677. Washington, D.C.: U.S. National Center for Health Statistics, 1968.

   Updates the earlier report on mortality and natality data (see no. 2.2). Also contains tables and life expectancy, marriages, and divorces not covered in the earlier volume.

2.2   Lindner, Forrest E., and Grove, Robert D. VITAL STATISTICS RATES IN THE UNITED STATES, 1900-1940. Washington, D.C.: U.S. Bureau of the Census, 1943.

   Brings together and summarizes past trends of mortality and natality rates. Was intended as an aid and guide for health administrators and social analysts.

2.3   U.S. Bureau of Community Health Services. IMPROVEMENT IN INFANT AND PERINATAL MORTALITY IN THE UNITED STATES, 1965-1973. DHEW publication no. (HSA) 78-5743. Washington, D.C.: Government Printing Office, 1978.

   Identifies changes in infant and fetal mortality by age-at-death or length of gestation, race, and degree of urbanization. Latest available date from the U.S. National Center for Health Statistics. Excludes Puerto Rico, Virgin Islands, Guam, and trust territories. Discusses data sources and methods.

2.4   U.S. Bureau of the Census. BIRTH, STILLBIRTH, AND INFANT MORTALITY STATISTICS, 1915-1936. Washington, D.C.: Government Printing Office, 1917-38.

   Superseded by VITAL STATISTICS OF THE UNITED STATES (see no. 2.14). Presents detailed statistics on births, stillbirths, and infant mortality as well as rates for each in the United States. Tables present data by cities, counties, and rural areas; data for births by age of parents, county of origin, race, and cases of plural births. Data for stillbirths and infant mortality are presented in these variables also. Data were compiled from transcripts of birth, death, and stillbirth certificates received from states and territories included in the registration area each year.

2.5   _____. MORTALITY STATISTICS, 1900-1936. Washington, D.C.: Government Printing Office, 1906-37.

   Superseded by VITAL STATISTICS OF THE UNITED STATES (see no. 2.14). Presents detailed statistics on deaths and death rates in the United States. Tables present data by cities and rural areas, race, age, sex, and cause. Data compiled from transcripts of certificates of deaths received from states and

Vital Statistics

territories included in the death registration area each year. Introduction to the 1936 volume describes the growth of the registration area from 1880 to 1936, when all states and territories in the United States were included.

2.6   U.S. Center for Disease Control. MMWR: MORBIDITY AND MORTALITY WEEKLY REPORT. Washington, D.C.: Government Printing Office, 1952-- .

Presents incidence of specified notifiable diseases for each week for the United States and each state. Also special analyses of different topics in each issue. Annual summary with final figures for morbidity and mortality in final issue each year. Includes trends for last ten years.

2.7   U.S. Indian Health Service. INDIAN HEALTH TRENDS AND SERVICES. Rockville, Md.: 1970-- . Irregular.

Includes extensive data on Indian vital and health statistics as well as information about health services. Contains information from INDIAN VITAL STATISTICS, formerly a separate publication.

2.8   U.S. National Center for Health Statistics. DATA ON MORTALITY. Vital and Health Statistics Series, no. 20. Washington, D.C.: Government Printing Office, 1965-- . Irregular.

(See no. 1.89.)

2.9   _____. DATA ON NATALITY, MARRIAGE AND DIVORCE. Vital and Health Statistics Series, no. 21. Washington, D.C.: Government Printing Office, 1965-- . Irregular.

(See no. 1.89.)

2.10   _____. MONTHLY VITAL STATISTICS REPORT. Washington, D.C.: 1952-- .

Provisional statistics on births, marriages, divorces, and deaths. Gives tabular data for each month and same month a year ago, with cumulative totals for each of three years. Time lag of thirteen weeks for mortality data and eight weeks for other data.

2.11   _____. UNITED STATES DECENNIAL LIFE TABLES FOR 1969-71, VOL. II, NOS. 1-51: STATE LIFE TABLES. Washington, D.C.: Government Printing Office, 1976.

Contains detailed state life tables for 1969-71 that are part of the decennial life-table program which began with tables for 1900-1902.

Vital Statistics

2.12 _____. UNITED STATES LIFE TABLES, 1969-71. Vol 1, no. 1. DHEW publication no. (HRA) 75-1150. Washington, D.C.: Government Printing Office, 1976.

Gives current life tables for the United States based on age-specific mortality rates. Also contains information related to the decennial life-table program which began with tables for 1900-1902.

2.13 _____. VITAL STATISTICS ADVANCE DATA. Washington, D.C.: Government Printing Office, 1976-- .

Issues contain selected findings from health and demographic surveys conducted by NCHS. Provides a means for early release of data previously issued as supplements to the MONTHLY VITAL STATISTICS REPORT (see no. 2.10). MVSR supplements with provisional and final vital statistics will still be published.

2.14 _____. VITAL STATISTICS OF THE UNITED STATES. 3 vols. Washington, D.C.: Government Printing Office, 1937-- . Annual.

Supersedes U.S. Bureau of the Census MORTALITY STATISTICS (see no. 2.5) and BIRTH, STILLBIRTH, AND INFANT MORTALITY STATISTICS (see no. 2.4). Published in the following three volumes: Volume 1, NATALITY, contains summary tables showing trends in period and cohort fertility measures and characteristics of live births. Frequency tabulations for detailed geographic areas also shown. Volume 2, part A, MORTALITY, contains general, infant, fetal, and accident mortality statistics with demographic and cause of death detail. Includes annual life table. Volume 2, part B, MORTALITY, presents total number of deaths, deaths by selected causes, infant deaths, neonatal deaths, fetal deaths, and rates and ratios. Tabulations shown by each state and county, specified urban places, metropolitan, and nonmetropolitan areas as well as standard metropolitan statistical areas (SMSAs).

2.15 U.S. National Heart and Lung Institute. SMOKING AND GENERAL MORTALITY AMONG U.S. VETERANS, 1954-1969. Washington, D.C.: Government Printing Office, 1970.

Describes the general mortality experience as related to tobacco use of almost 300,000 U.S. veterans who held government life insurance policies in 1953 and have been followed for sixteen years.

2.16 U.S. National Institute for Occupational Safety and Health. OCCUPATIONAL MORTALITY IN WASHINGTON STATE, 1950-1971. Washington, D.C.: Government Printing Office, 1976.

Vital Statistics

Gives detailed cause of death analysis (160 cases) for each of 194 occupational classes. Compares mortality findings with those of the other U.S. study, VITAL STATISTICS--SPECIAL REPORTS, vol. 53, no. 3, 1963 (see no. 1.88).

Chapter 3
MORBIDITY

Illness or morbidity can be divided into two general categories--communicable and chronic. Communicable diseases are reportable by law while chronic diseases are not. This chapter provides references to serials and monographs covering the two types of morbidity.

The publications have been divided into two major sections. The first contains references to the major surveillance series covering communicable diseases and chronic conditions; the second contains references to specific diseases and other health-related problems.

SERIES

The surveillance of communicable disease is chiefly the responsibility of the U.S. Center for Disease Control which publishes both the MORBIDITY AND MORTALITY WEEKLY REPORT (see no. 3.1) and the SURVEILLANCE REPORTS (see no. 3.2).

The collection of data concerning chronic diseases has been conducted mainly by the U.S. National Center for Health Statistics. The HEALTH EXAMINATION SURVEY (see no. 3.3) and the HEALTH INTERVIEW SURVEY (see no. 3.4) provide the most comprehensive data on chronic illnesses, although they are basically sample surveys providing national and regional estimates.

Data on chronic conditions for smaller than national or regional areas is one of the most sought-after, but poorly covered areas of health statistics.

3.1   U.S. Center for Disease Control. MMWR: MORBIDITY AND MORTALITY WEEKLY REPORT. Washington, D.C.: Government Printing Office, 1952-- .

   (See no. 2.6.)

Morbidity

3.2 _____. SURVEILLANCE REPORTS. Atlanta, Ga.: N.d. Irregular.

> Series of reports on a variety of communicable diseases and other issues in public health such as abortion. CDC receives data from state and local health departments, virology laboratories, and other "pertinent sources." Covers the following topics at the present time: diphtheria; foodborne disease (including botulism and waterborne); hepatitis; influenza; respiratory disease; malaria; measles; rubella; mumps; encephalitis; salmonellosis; shigellosis; trichinosis; rabies; abortion; congenital malformations; poliomyelitis; aseptic meningitis; national nosocomial infections study; veterinary public health; morbidity and mortality; brucellosis; leptospirosis; psittacosis; Rh hemolytic disease; and enterovirus disease.

3.3 U.S. National Center for Health Statistics. DATA FROM THE HEALTH EXAMINATION SURVEY. Vital and Health Statistics Series, no. 11. Washington, D.C.: Government Printing Office, 1964-- . Irregular.

> Series of reports based on examining and testing selected individuals from a population sample. Includes estimates of the prevalence of selected chronic diseases and other health indicators. Provide national and regional estimates only.

3.4 _____. DATA FROM THE HEALTH INTERVIEW SURVEY. Vital and Health Statistics Series no. 10. Washington, D.C.: Government Printing Office, 1963-- . Irregular.

> Series of reports based on a periodic sample survey of households. Provide national and regional estimates for a variety of disabilities, acute conditions, and utilization of health services.

3.5 World Health Organization. WEEKLY EPIDEMILOGICAL RECORD. Geneva: 1947-- .

> Prepared for the guidance of health administrators and health authorities, contains epidemiological surveillance data of communicable diseases throughout the world. Notes on different diseases with a list of newly affected areas in each issue.

SPECIFIC DISEASES AND HEALTH CONDITIONS

There are a variety of sources for data on diseases, some public and some private. They do not, however, cover all the diseases one might imagine. Chronic diseases, disabilities, and other nonreportable health conditions present difficulties in collection, especially for incidence data. Prevalance data is more likely to be available. The U.S. National Center for Health Statistics Surveys (see nos. 3.3 and 3.4) mentioned in the previous section provide coverage for the greatest number of diseases. Other agencies or organizations who gather data generally concentrate on one disease.

Morbidity

Noteworthy are the publications of the various national institutes of health (see nos. 3.18-3.24 and no. 3.27). Private organizations such as the American Cancer Society (see no. 3.13) and the National Health Education Committee (see no. 3.57) also provide information.

Data on the incidence and prevalence of specific diseases may be found in journal literature, accessible through the various indexes, abstracts, and online services described in chapter 1. The statistics, however, may apply only to a small sample of the population on which a study was based.

Accidents and Injuries

3.6 Bunker, J.P., et al. THE NATIONAL HALOTHANE STUDY. Bethesda, Md.: National Institute of General Medical Sciences, 1969.

   A study of the use of halothane anesthesia and postoperative hepatitis as well as other anesthetic agents and postoperative mortality. Data on age, sex, physical status of patient, and type of anesthesia used.

3.7 Consumer Product Safety Commission. NEISS NEWS. Washington, D.C.: 1972-- . Monthly.

   Data from the National Electronic Injury Surveillance System. Consists of 119 hospital emergency rooms participating in NEISS. Bases data tables on the ninety product categories in the Consumer Product Hazard Index.

3.8 National Safety Council. ACCIDENT FACTS. Chicago: 1972-- . Annual.

   Presents detailed analysis of accidents, including motor vehicle, work, home, and public. Analyses include: costs of accidents, accident deaths vs. other causes of death, and trends in accidental death rates. Includes tables with geographic breakdowns.

3.9 U.S. Food and Drug Administration. National Clearinghouse for Poison Control Centers. POISON CONTROL STATISTICS. Rockville, Md.: 1968-- . Annual.

   Compiles reports of individual cases to the poison control centers. Data describe product type and brand, victim's age and symptoms, and circumstances of the incident.

Alcoholism

3.10 Efron, Vera; Keller, Mark; and Guriolo, C. STATISTICS ON CONSUMPTION OF ALCOHOL AND ALCOHOLISM. New Brunswick, N.J.: Rutgers University, 1974.

Morbidity

3.11   U.S. National Institute on Alcohol Abuse and Alcoholism. THIRD SPECIAL REPORT TO THE U.S. CONGRESS ON ALCOHOL AND HEALTH. DHEW publication no. (ADM) 78-569. Washington, D.C.: Government Printing Office, 1978.

> Contains tables throughout the narrative presenting data on: (1) alcohol consumption among teenagers, adults, and older persons (by state, region, seventeen foreign countries, and beverage) by sex; (2) economic costs; (3) health effects-- statistical correlations between alcohol and disease; (4) traffic accidents. Updates first and second special report.

Botulism

3.12   U.S. Center for Disease Control. BOTULISM IN THE UNITED STATES, 1899-1973. Atlanta, Ga.: 1974.

> Reviews the epidemiology of botulism in the United States since 1899, the problems of clinical and laboratory diagnosis, and current concepts of treatment.

Cancer

3.13   American Cancer Society. CANCER FACTS AND FIGURES. New York: 19?-- . Annual.

> Compilation of basic data regarding cancer including incidence, survival, mortality, and trends. Some data by state, but generally for the United States as a whole.

3.14   Bridbord, Kenneth, et al. ESTIMATES OF THE FRACTION OF CANCER IN THE UNITED STATES RELATED TO OCCUPATIONAL DISEASES. Bethesda, Md.: National Cancer Institute, National Institute of Environmental Health Sciences and National Institute for Occupational Safety and Health, 1978.

> Paper which addresses occupationally related cancers with estimates and comparisons throughout. Compares asbestos risks with those due to five other substances and smoking. Includes tables showing chemicals associated with cancer in man and estimated numbers of workers exposed. Also tells occupational groups in which excess cancer incidence has been reported. Cites important epidemiological studies in large bibliography.

3.15   Doll, Richard. CANCER INCIDENCE IN FIVE CONTINENTS. 2 vols. New York: Springer, 1966-70.

> Data contributed for first volume from the cancer registries in twenty-four countries; second volume reports data for fifty-eight populations. Volumes bring together available cancer incidence

Morbidity

data in one place and present the data in the same way so that researchers can make whatever comparisons they choose. A third volume was published in 1976 (see no. 3.25).

3.16 Macdonald, Eleanor J., and Heinze, Evelyn B. EPIDEMIOLOGY OF CANCER IN TEXAS: INCIDENCE ANALYZED BY TYPE, ETHNIC GROUP, AND GEOGRAPHIC LOCATION. New York: Raven Press, 1978.

Presents detailed information on cancer incidence by site for six large regions (fifty-six counties) in Texas. Covers a twenty-three-year period and three ethnic groups (white, nonwhite, and Spanish surname) in a population of four million. Every medical facility and every patient record during 1944-66 was inspected. Tables show age-adjusted and age-specific incidence rates per hundred-thousand population by ethnic group. Important study of incidence among various populations in varying environments.

3.17 Silverberg, Edwin. LEUKEMIAS AND LYMPHOMAS: STATISTICAL AND EPIDEMIOLOGICAL INFORMATION. New York: American Cancer Society, 1977.

Provides data on incidence, probability, mortality, treatment, and survival for leukemia, Hodgkin's disease, reticulosarcoma, lymphosarcoma, multiple myeloma, and other neoplasm of the blood and lymph systems. Has 223 references to other epidemiological studies.

3.18 U.S. National Cancer Institute. ATLAS OF CANCER MORTALITY AMONG U.S. NONWHITES, 1950-69. DHEW publication no. (NIH) 76-1204. Washington, D.C.: Government Printing Office, 1976.

Maps based on compilations of cancer deaths and age-adjusted death rates by sex and race. Presents data for cancer mortality by the five major racial groups--whites, blacks, American Indians, Chinese, and Japanese.

3.19 _____. ATLAS OF CANCER MORTALITY FOR U.S. COUNTIES, 1950-1969. By Thomas J. Mason. DHEW publication no. (NIH) 75-780. Bethesda, Md.: 1975.

Atlas shows geographic variation in cancer death rates across the United States for thirty-five anatomic sites of cancer. Contains maps of sixteen common cancer sites on a county-by-county basis; other nineteen sites by state economic area (SEA). Survivor tables for each cancer site follow maps, listing a percentile ranking of both mortality rates and numbers of deaths.

Morbidity

3.20 _____. U.S. CANCER MORTALITY BY COUNTY, 1950-69. DHEW publication no. NIH 74-615. Washington, D.C.: Government Printing Office, 1974.

Presents for each county in the United States cancer deaths and age-adjusted death rates according to sex and race over a twenty-year period.

3.21 U.S. National Cancer Institute. Biometry Branch. CANCER RATES AND RISKS. 2d ed. DHEW publication no. (NIH) 74-691. Washington, D.C.: Government Printing Office, 1974.

Presents information on the measurable aspects of cancer, including variations and trends in cancer incidence and mortality. Also gives some aspects of diagnosis and treatment, survival rates for diagnosed cancer cases, and prospects for future progress.

3.22 _____. THIRD NATIONAL CANCER SURVEY--ADVANCED THREE-YEAR REPORT, 1969-71 INCIDENCE. DHEW publication no. (NIH) 74-637. Washington, D.C.: Government Printing Office, 1974.

Provides incidence data for the years 1969 through 1971 for seven metropolitan areas and two entire states. Contains figures for the resident cases of cancer newly diagnosed during the three years.

3.23 U.S. National Cancer Institute. End Results Section. CANCER PATIENT SURVIVAL. Washington, D.C.: Government Printing Office. no. 5-- . 1977-- .

Previous title: END RESULTS IN CANCER, report nos. 1-4, 1950-73. A series of comprehensive reports on the survival of cancer patients. Analysis of data with respect to age, race, sex, primary site, cell type, extent of disease, and treatment. No. 5 provides data for the period 1950-73. Issues titled END RESULTS IN CANCER provide data for 1940-50.

3.24 _____. TREATMENT AND SURVIVAL PATTERNS FOR BLACK AND WHITE CANCER PATIENTS, 1955-1964. By Lillian M. Axtell. DHEW publication no. (NIH) 75-712. Washington, D.C.: Government Printing Office, 1975.

The first comprehensive report issued by the Biometry Branch of the U.S. National Cancer Institute which evaluates the end results of cancer among black and white patients. Presents data for twenty-eight sites of primary cancer.

Morbidity

3.25   Waterhouse, J., et al. CANCER INCIDENCE IN FIVE CONTINENTS. Vol. 3. IARC Scientific Publication no. 15. Lyon, France: International Agency for Research on Cancer, 1976.

> Data from cancer registries throughout the world. Editors indicate reliability of the data. Tables present data by age-specific incidence rates for Africa, America, Asia, Europe, and Oceania and Australia. Includes index to World Health publications which have cancer statistics and a cumulated index for volumes 1, 2, and 3. (See no. 3.15 for volumes 1 and 2.)

Diabetes

3.26   U.S. National Commission on Diabetes. REPORT OF THE NATIONAL COMMISSION ON DIABETES TO THE CONGRESS OF THE UNITED STATES. 4 vols. Bethesda, Md.: National Institutes of Health, 1976.

> Comprehensive report on the incidence and prevalence of diabetes by age, geographic, and sex variables. Statistics also on diseases associated with diabetes such as ocular and renal disease, coronary heart disease, neuropathy, and coma. Includes extensive data on the economic impact of diabetes with data on the cost of diabetes in terms of direct and indirect costs.

3.27   U.S. National Institute of Arthritis, Metabolism and Digestive Diseases. DIABETES DATA. DHEW publication no. (NIH) 78-1468. Washington, D.C.: Government Printing Office, 1978.

> Compilation of facts ranging from clinical information to the socioeconomic impact of the disease. Statistical scope includes incidence and prevalence data, morbidity of long- and short-term complications, and diabetes mortality.

Disability

3.28   U.S. Social Security Administration. DISABILITY SURVEY 71: RECENTLY DISABLED ADULTS. DHEW publication no. (SSA) 76-11716. Washington, D.C.: Government Printing Office, 1976.

> Data collected from about 1,400 noninstitutionalized adults identified as disabled in 1971. Reports focus on analysis of factors associated with the disability such as income, health, and social consequences for the disabled person.

3.29   _____. DISABILITY SURVEY 72: DISABLED AND NON-DISABLED ADULTS. DHEW publication no. (SSA) 77-11717. Washington, D.C.: Government Printing Office, 1977.

Morbidity

Data collected from about 18,000 disabled, nondisabled, and previously disabled adults in 1972. Reports focus on the socioeconomic standing of the disabled person and his family. Also compares medical charges for the disabled and the nondisabled.

Drug Abuse

3.30   U.S. National Institute on Drug Abuse. DATA FROM THE CLIENT ORIENTED DATA ACQUISITION PROCESS (CODAP), SERIES E. Rockville, Md.: 1975-- . Annual.

Annual report on the characteristics of clients admitted to and discharged from federally funded drug abuse treatment programs. Shows percent distribution of clients by drugs of abuse, mode of treatment, and treatment facility.

3.31   _____. DATA FROM THE NATIONAL DRUG ABUSE TREATMENT UTILIZATION SURVEY (NDATUS), SERIES F. Rockville, Md.: 1976-- . Irregular.

Series of reports on the characteristics, utilization, staff, and funding of drug abuse treatment services, public and private.

3.32   _____. DRUG USE AMONG AMERICAN HIGH SCHOOL STUDENTS. Rockville, Md.: 1975-1977-- . Annual.

First annual report on the prevalence and frequency of illicit drug use by high school seniors. Includes data from three annual surveys of fifteen thousand seniors 1975-77. Research conducted by the Institute for Social Research, University of Michigan. Drugs include: marihuana, inhalants, hallucinogens, cocaine, heroin, other opiates, stimulants, sedatives, tranquilizers, alcohol, and cigarettes. Also considers attitudes toward drug use and trends in drug use.

3.33   _____. HEROIN INDICATORS TREND REPORT. DHEW publication no. (ADM) 76-315. Washington, D.C.: Government Printing Office, 1976-- . Irregular.

Reports provide an objective assessment of heroin indicator trend data in this country. Indicators include: (1) medical examiner reports on drug-related deaths, (2) emergency room reports on drug-related episodes, (3) hepatitis reports, (4) reports on the drug retail price and purity levels, (5) state and local law enforcement reports on drug law arrests, (6) drug abuse treatment program admission records. The reports focus on patterns of heroin use. Gives sources of data and brief bibliographies.

Morbidity

3.34 _____. MARIHUANA AND HEALTH: ANNUAL REPORT TO THE U.S. CONGRESS FROM THE SECRETARY OF HEALTH, EDUCATION, AND WELFARE. Washington, D.C.: Government Printing Office, 1971-- . Annual.

Reviews research on marihuana use and its health consequences. Contains tables on the nature and extent of use among adults and teenagers by age and sex. Also some figures and trends in its use.

3.35 _____. NATIONAL SURVEY OF DRUG ABUSE. 3 vols. Washington, D.C.: Government Printing Office, 1977-- . Annual.

Earlier volumes for 1971, 1972, 1974-75 published only by contractor. Available on microfiche from National Technical Information Service. The 1975-76 volume titled NONMEDICAL USE OF PSYCHOACTIVE SUBSTANCES (see no. 3.36). Reports based on a national probability sample of adolescents and adults from a household survey. Data on prevalence and frequency of illegal drug use, medical and nonmedical use of prescription drugs.

3.36 _____. NONMEDICAL USE OF PSYCHOACTIVE SUBSTANCES: 1975-76 NATIONWIDE STUDY AMONG YOUTH AND ADULTS. Washington, D.C.: 1976.

Data from a national sample include a study of experience with and beliefs about a wide range of legal and illicit drugs. Covers (1) glue and other inhalants, (2) LSD and other hallucinogens, and (3) opiates. Data questions include reasons used and frequency of use.

3.37 _____. YOUNG MEN AND DRUGS: A NATIONWIDE SURVEY. NIDA Research Monograph 5. Washington, D.C.: Government Printing Office, 1976.

Presents mainly prevalence data on drug abuse among young men aged twenty to thirty years in 1974. Includes use of the following drugs: tobacco, alcohol, marihuana, psychedelics, stimulants, sedatives, heroin, opiates, and cocaine.

Epilepsy

3.38 U.S. Commission for the Control of Epilepsy and Its Consequences. PLAN FOR NATIONWIDE ACTION ON EPILEPSY. Vol. 4. Bethesda, Md.: U.S. National Institute of Neurological, Communicative Disorders and Stroke, 1977.

Study examines medical and social problems of epilepsy. Volume 4, EPIDEMIOLOGY AND ECONOMICS OF EPILEPSY (NIH 78-279), presents data on incidence, prevalence, prognosis and

Morbidity

mortality. Economic data include estimates of losses from unemployment and excess mortality, costs of treatment, rehabilitation and research. Also estimate numbers of neurologists needed to provide medical care to epileptics 1975-2000.

Heart Disease

3.39   U.S. National Heart and Lung Institute. THE FRAMINGHAM STUDY: AN EPIDEMIOLOGICAL INVESTIGATION OF CARDIOVASCULAR DISEASE. Washington, D.C.: Government Printing Office, 1968-- . Irregular.

Reports present data of a longitudinal study to determine the appearance of cardiovascular disease in a sample of the adult population of Framingham, Massachusetts. Follows subjects aged between thirty and fifty-nine for twenty years, beginning in 1948, through ten clinical examinations given in two-year intervals. Thirty-two sections published to date.

Hypertension

3.40   _____. THE PUBLIC AND HIGH BLOOD PRESSURE. DHEW publication no. (NIH) 74-356. Washington, D.C.: Government Printing Office, 1973.

A poll conducted by Harris and Associates. Provides information on what the public knows about hypertension, what it does about it, and the effects it has had on the life-style of individuals. Broken into age, sex, and race categories.

Mental Health

3.41   U.S. National Institute of Mental Health. REPORT SERIES ON MENTAL HEALTH STATISTICS. Washington, D.C.: Government Printing Office, 1969-- . Irregular.

Series A--MENTAL HEALTH FACILITIES REPORTS. Descriptive data on facilities, patients served, staffing, and expenditures, 1969-- .
Series B--ANALYTICAL AND SPECIAL STUDY REPORTS. Special purpose studies or detailed analytical and interpretive reports, 1969-- .
Series C--METHODOLOGY REPORTS. New statistical methodology, data collection techniques, 1969-- .
Series D--CONFERENCE OR COMMITTEE REPORTS AND ANALYTICAL REVIEW OF LITERATURE. Subjects of general interest to the field, 1970-- .

3.42   _____. STATISTICAL NOTES. Rockville, Md.: 1969-- . Irregular.

Morbidity

Brief presentations of data dealing with specific topics such as educational level of admissions to state mental hospitals, accessibility of community mental health centers, and length of stay in general hospital psychiatric inpatient units. Content usually includes tabular presentations and highlights of data.

Nutrition

3.43 U.S. Center for Disease Control. Nutrition Program. TEN-STATE NUTRITION SURVEY, 1968-1970. DHEW publication no. (HSM) 72-8130. Atlanta, Ga.: 1972.

Survey collected five types of data: general demographic, dietary intake, clinical, dental, and biochemical, from ten states representative of their geographic region and New York City.

3.44 U.S. National Center for Health Statistics. PRELIMINARY FINDINGS OF THE FIRST HEALTH AND NUTRITION EXAMINATION SURVEY, UNITED STATES, 1971-72: ANTHROPOMETRIC AND CLINICAL FINDINGS. DHEW publication no. (HRA) 75-1229. Washington, D.C.: Government Printing Office, 1975.

Findings collected on a probability sample of the U.S. population by age, sex, race, and income level, 1971-72. Presents data on selected anthropometric measurements of children one to seventeen years of age, obesity in adults twenty to seventy-four years of age, and clinical signs of nutritional deficiency for persons one to seventy-four years of age.

3.45 _____. PRELIMINARY FINDINGS OF THE FIRST HEALTH AND NUTRITION EXAMINATION SURVEY, UNITED STATES, 1971-72: DIETARY INTAKE AND BIOCHEMICAL FINDINGS. DHEW publication no. (HRA) 74-1219. Washington, D.C.: Government Printing Office, 1974.

Presents preliminary findings on the dietary intake and biochemical levels of various nutrients in a probability sample of U.S. population one to seventy-four years of age, by age, sex, race, and income level, 1971-72.

Occupational Health

3.46 U.S. Bureau of Labor Statistics. OCCUPATIONAL INJURIES AND ILLNESSES IN THE UNITED STATES, BY INDUSTRY. BLS Bulletin. Washington, D.C.: Government Printing Office, 1972-- . Annual.

Annual report on occupational injuries and illnesses for the private sector by detailed industry. Data reported by large sample of all firms covered by the Occupational Health and

Morbidity

Safety Act of 1970. Covers incidence rates and average workdays lost. Previous reports contained data by state, 1972-74. State data will be published separately starting with 1975 data.

3.47 U.S. National Institute for Occupational Safety and Health. HEALTH AND WORK IN AMERICA: APHA CHARTBOOK. Washington, D.C.: Government Printing Office, 1975.

Compilation of charts on occupationally related health and safety of U.S. workers prepared by American Public Health Association under contract.

Smoking

3.48 U.S. Center for Disease Control. CHARTBOOK ON SMOKING, TOBACCO, AND HEALTH. DHEW publication no. (CDC) 76-8718. Washington, D.C.: Government Printing Office, 1976.

Charts and tables on smoking and health, as well as tables on cigarettes and the economy.

3.49 U.S. National Clearinghouse for Smoking and Health. ADULT USE OF TOBACCO--1975. Atlanta, Ga.: 1976.

Data on smokers includes demographic information, attitudes towards smoking and health, smoking history, and dosage. Focuses on cigarettes, but includes some data on other forms of tobacco. Data for studies conducted in 1964, 1966, and 1970 available from CDC.

Tuberculosis

3.50 U.S. Center for Disease Control. TUBERCULOSIS IN THE UNITED STATES. Publication no. (CDC) 76-8322. Atlanta, Ga.: 1976.

Incorporates statistics previously published separately in REPORTED TUBERCULOSIS DATA AND TUBERCULOSIS PROGRAMS and is a companion report to TUBERCULOSIS STATISTICS: STATES AND CITIES (see no. 3.52). Reviews tuberculosis morbidity and mortality and presents an analysis of the current status of the disease in the United States. Data submitted to CDC by state and city health departments.

3.51 _____. TUBERCULOSIS IN THE WORLD. By Anthony N. Lowell. DHEW publication no. (CDC) 76-8317. Washington, D.C.: Government Printing Office, 1976.

Report on tuberculosis morbidity and mortality throughout the world covering 1950-74. Data from World Health Organization

Morbidity

and other foreign statistical publications. Countries are arranged by world region; data for each when available include number of cases, case rates, death rates, and breakdown by form of disease, age, and sex.

3.52 _____. TUBERCULOSIS STATISTICS: STATES AND CITIES. Atlanta, Ga.: 1970-- . Annual.

Shows new tuberculosis cases and case rates as reported by state and city health departments and tuberculosis beds in hospitals based on CDC surveys. Cases shown by age, sex, and race.

Venereal Disease

3.53 U.S. Center for Disease Control. SEXUALLY TRANSMITTED DISEASE (STD) STATISTICAL LETTER. Washington, D.C.: Government Printing Office, 1978-- . Semiannual.

Formerly VD STATISTICAL LETTER. Tabulates venereal disease cases reported to the U.S. Public Health Service by state and territorial health departments. Shows cases and rates by state, region, and city.

3.54 _____. STD FACT SHEET. Atlanta, Ga.: 1978-- . Annual.

Formerly VD FACT SHEET (1943-78). Summarizes incidence and prevalence of syphilis and gonorrhea as well as historical trends. Data collected by CDC for state and local health departments.

Vision and Hearing

3.55 Kahn, H.A., and Moorhead, H.B. STATISTICS ON BLINDNESS IN THE MODEL REPORTING AREA, 1968-70. DHEW publication no. (NIH) 73-427. Washington, D.C.: Government Printing Office, 1973.

The model reporting area consisted of fourteen states in which the registered blind were reported. Gives statistics on blindness by etiology as well as by sex, race, and age variables for each state and for the total area. The first model reporting area statistics covered 1966 and 1968. Discontinued.

3.56 Schein, Jerome D. THE DEAF POPULATION OF THE UNITED STATES. Silver Spring, Md.: National Association of the Deaf, 1974.

Provides an estimate of the size and geographical distribution of the deaf population and gives selected characteristics of people with hearing impairments. Includes many tables.

Morbidity

Miscellaneous

3.57   National Health Education Committee. THE KILLERS AND CRIPPLERS: FACTS ON MAJOR DISEASE IN THE UNITED STATES TODAY. 11th ed. New York: David McKay, 1976.

Covers many chronic diseases, for further discussion see no. 1.8.

3.57a   U.S. Bureau of Community Health Services. HEALTH STATUS OF CHILDREN: A REVIEW OF SURVEYS 1963-1972. DHEW publication no. (HSA) 78-5744. Washington, D.C.: Government Printing Office, 1978.

A followup to the 1963 Children's Bureau publication ILLNESS AMONG CHILDREN. Examines acute and chronic illnesses among children, dental care, and disparities in health care for children of minority and low-income families. Also includes nutrition. Major data sources from NCHS ongoing surveys: (1) Health Interview Survey, (2) Health Examination Survey, (3) Health and Nutrition Examination Survey, and (4) Hospital Discharge Survey. Other findings taken from: (1) Ten-State Nutrition Survey, (2) Study of Nutritional Status of Preschool Children in the U.S., 1968-70, and (3) Adolescent Health in Harlem. Summarizes each survey separately with many charts and tables. Compares more recent findings to the studies done fifteen years earlier in the final chapter.

3.58   U.S. Indian Health Service. ILLNESS AMONG INDIANS, 1965-69. DHEW publication no. (HSM) 72-507. Washington, D.C.: Government Printing Office, 1971.

Summarizes notifiable disease data for five years. Includes a brief description of demographic characteristics of Indian and Alaska native populations.

3.59   U.S. Public Health Service. Federal Security Agency. ILLNESS AND MEDICAL CARE AMONG 2,500,000 PERSONS IN 83 CITIES WITH SPECIAL REFERENCE TO SOCIO-ECONOMIC FACTORS. Washington, D.C.: Government Printing Office, 1945.

Collection of papers on illness and medical care based on the National Health Survey of 1935-36. Survey included studies of (1) disabling illness, (2) chronic diseases, (3) medical care, (4) accidents, (5) orthopedic impairments, (6) blindness, (7) diseases of childhood, (8) housing, (9) fertility, and (10) population. Included in this bibliography for purposes of historical comparison.

3.60   U.S. Veterans Administration. THE MOST FREQUENTLY OCCURRING DIAGNOSES IN VA HOSPITALS, 1971-1976. Controller Monograph 4. Washington, D.C.: Government Printing Office, 1977.

Morbidity

Statistics concerning the frequencies of diagnostic condition for which patients were hospitalized and treated in VA hospitals during 1971-77. Counts all diagnoses reported in any episode of care. Omits patients treated and diagnosed as outpatients.

Chapter 4
HEALTH RESOURCES

Listed in this chapter are sources which provide statistics on health resources. The sources have been divided into three sections: (1) Health Facilities, (2) Health Manpower, and (3) Health Education.

HEALTH FACILITIES

Sources of health facility data include both public and private organizations. Inadequacies of the data available include incomplete coverage of all types of facilities, but most notably outpatient facilities and long-term care facilities.

The major source of data from the public sector is the U.S. National Center for Health Statistics which publishes several statistical reports from data in its MASTER FACILITIES INVENTORY. This inventory includes hospitals, nursing homes and other inpatient facilities (see nos. 4.4, 4.5, 4.6, 4.7).

The American Hospital Association is the major publisher of data on hospitals and other facilities in its annual GUIDE TO THE HEALTH CARE FIELD (see no. 4.2).

4.1   American Hospital Association. COMPARATIVE STATISTICS ON HEALTH FACILITIES AND POPULATION; METROPOLITAN AND NONMETROPOLITAN AREAS. Chicago: 1978.

4.2   _____. GUIDE TO THE HEALTH CARE FIELD. Chicago: 1945-- . Annual.

   Central reference source for information on health care institutions. Includes hospitals and long-term care facilities registered by the association as health facilities. Data for each institution includes services offered, accreditation status, ownership, membership status, number of beds, admissions, occupancy rate, address and telephone numbers, number of personnel, and name of administrator. Also gives educational programs in the health care field and sources of products and services for hospitals.

Health Resources

4.3 U.S. Health Resources Administration. DIRECTORY OF NURSING HOME FACILITIES. 5 vols. DHEW publication nos. (HRA) 72-20001-20005. Washington, D.C.: Government Printing Office, 1975.

> Covers geographic regions--West, Northeastern, North Central, Southern, and Western. Includes number of beds for each facility along with names and addresses of nursing homes from 1973. Arranged alphabetically by city within state.

4.4 U.S. National Center for Health Statistics. DATA ON HEALTH RESOURCES: MANPOWER AND FACILITIES. Vital and Health Statistics Series, no. 14. Washington, D.C.: Government Printing Office, 1963-- . Irregular.

> Statistics on the numbers, geographic distribution, and characteristics of health resources including physicians, dentists, nurses, other health occupations, hospitals, nursing homes, and outpatient facilities.

4.5 _____. HEALTH RESOURCES STATISTICS: HEALTH MANPOWER AND FACILITIES. 1976-77 ed. DHEW publication no. (PHS) 79-1509. Washington, D.C.: Government Printing Office, 1979.

> Provides current and comprehensive statistics on a wide range of health areas as baseline data for the planning, administration and evaluation of health programs. Statistics for occupations designated as "health occupations, including allied health occupations" in part 1. Statistics on facilities designated as "inpatient health facilities" in part 2. Statistics on "outpatient and nonpatient health services" in part 3.

4.6 _____. HOSPITALS: A COUNTY AND METROPOLITAN AREA DATA BOOK, 1974. By Genevieve W. Strahon. PHS publication no. 78-1223. Washington, D.C.: Government Printing Office, 1977.

> Includes hospitals by type, number of beds, and staff by state. Lists beds, average daily census, and ownership of general and specialty hospitals for SMSA's.

4.7 _____. NURSING HOMES--A COUNTY AND METROPOLITAN AREA DATA BOOK. DHEW publication no. (HSM) 73-1215. Washington, D.C.: Government Printing Office, 1976.

> Data by SMSA and by county for all states in the United States. Tabulates number of homes, number of beds, number of residents, personnel, and occupancy rate. Separates information on homes providing nursing care from that of homes not providing nursing care.

Health Resources

4.8   U.S. National Institute of Mental Health. MENTAL HEALTH FACILITIES REPORTS. REPORT SERIES ON MENTAL HEALTH STATISTICS, SERIES A. Washington, D.C.: Government Printing Office, 1969-- . Irregular.

   Include descriptive data on facilities, patients served, staffing, and expenditures.

HEALTH MANPOWER

The situation for health manpower statistics is similar to that for health facilities. Both public and private agencies collect and publish data, not really covering the field completely. Major sources of health manpower data are professional organizations such as the American Medical Association (see no. 4.12), the American Dental Association (see no. 4.11), and the American Nurses' Association (see no. 4.14).

Significant studies of health manpower have been made by the U.S. Health Resources Administration and its major components, for example, the Bureau of Health Manpower and Resources Development and the Bureau of Health Manpower. The U.S. National Center for Health Statistics also provides information on an ongoing basis in its publications series (see no. 4.4).

4.9   Altenfelder, Marion. MINORITIES AND WOMEN IN THE HEALTH FIELDS: APPLICANTS, STUDENTS, AND WORKERS. DHEW publication no. (HRA) 76-22. Health Manpower References. Washington, D.C.: Government Printing Office, 1979.

   Divided into two parts. Contains tables with information by racial and ethnic category in the first part and tables with information by sex in the second part. Gives data for the following health occupations: medicine, osteopathic medicine, dentistry, optometry, pharmacy, podiatry, veterinary medicine, nursing, allied health, and public health (part 2 only).

4.10   _____. OSTEOPATHIC PHYSICIANS IN THE UNITED STATES: A REPORT ON A 1971 SURVEY. NTIS PB-243 439/AS. Springfield, Va.: National Technical Information Service, 1975.

   Presents data about osteopathic physicians by age, sex, year of graduation, federal and nonfederal, and specialty, for both the United States and individual states.

4.11   American Dental Association. DISTRIBUTION OF DENTISTS IN THE UNITED STATES BY STATE, REGION, DISTRICT AND COUNTY, 1976. Chicago: 1977-- . Annual.

   Includes data on retired dentists, specialists, foreign dentists, and women dentists.

Health Resources

4.12 American Medical Association. Center for Health Research and Development. PHYSICIAN DISTRIBUTION AND MEDICAL LICENSURE IN THE UNITED STATES. Chicago: 1974-- . Annual.

Supersedes DISTRIBUTION OF PHYSICIANS IN THE UNITED STATES, 1963-73. A standard work which provides information on the geographic distribution of medical practice in the United States and possessions. Serves as a guide for comparing regions, divisions, states, and counties with respect to their total number of physicians by specialty and professional activity; number of hospitals and hospital beds; number of inhabitants, some general economic characteristics. Includes statistics dealing with medical licensure in the United States beginning with this edition. Part 1--physician distribution by regional, state, county, and metropolitan areas; Part 2--annual report of medical licensure statistics.

4.13 _____. REFERENCE DATA ON THE PROFILE OF MEDICAL PRACTICE. Chicago: 1971-- . Annual.

(See no. 1.94.)

4.14 American Nurses' Association. FACTS ABOUT NURSING. New York: 1935-- . Annual.

The "authoritative source of fundamental nursing statistics." Presents data on nurse distribution, nursing education, and the economic status of registered nurses. Gives similar data for allied nursing personnel (LPN's, aids, and orderlies). Includes health facilities and utilization, expenditures for health care, and a summary of vital statistics of the United States.

4.15 Arnoff, Franklyn N., and Kumbor, A.H. THE NATION'S PSYCHIATRISTS--1970 SURVEY. Washington, D.C.: American Psychiatric Association, 1973.

Third report in a series of manpower studies made by the APA and NIMH. Organizes survey data into five categories starting with chapter 2, supply and demographic characteristics of the sample; chapter 3, education and training by sex, also data on FMG's; chapter 4, professional activities; chapter 5, geographic distribution by state per 100,000 population; chapter 6, economic issues, but no discussion of actual income.

4.16 Goodman, Louis J. THE SUPPLY AND AVAILABILITY OF PHYSICIAN SERVICES. Chicago: American Medical Association, 1977.

Shows historical trends and projections of physician supply from 1963 forward. Shows availability of services measured in terms of fulltime equivalents (FTE) by state for all specialties, general and family practitioners, and medical specialties on maps.

Health Resources

4.17   Hudson, Helen H. SOURCEBOOK: NURSING PERSONNEL. DHEW publication no. (HRA) 75-43. Health Manpower References. Washington, D.C.: Government Printing Office, 1975.

Contains historical and current statistics, references on the supply of nursing personnel, and potential resources for the nation. Data on registered and practical nurses including numbers distribution, licensure training, and field of practice.

4.18   Jolly, H.P. PARTICIPATION OF WOMEN AND MINORITIES ON U.S. MEDICAL SCHOOL FACULTIES. Washington, D.C.: American Association of Medical Colleges, 1976.

Data on the distribution of medical school faculty by sex, ethnic group, degree, and department. Gives trends and the percentage of females for each category.

4.19   Knopf, Lucille. RN'S ONE AND FIVE YEARS AFTER GRADUATION. New York: National League for Nursing, 1975.

Part of the nurse-career pattern study by the National League for Nursing which is to follow the same cohorts for a period of fifteen years at selected intervals after graduation. Presents data for one-year and five-year graduates by type of nursing program with the following variables: marital status, work status, changes of employment, education, licensure, and professional activities.

4.20   U.S. Bureau of Health Manpower. OPTOMETRIC MANPOWER RESOURCES, 1973. DHEW publication no. (HRA) 76-101. Washington, D.C.: Government Printing Office, 1976.

Report on the number of optometrists licensed to practice in the United States, 1973. Covers race and ethnicity, school of graduation, and state and region of practice. Based on a 1973 survey of 19,541 optometrists conducted by the International Association of Boards of Examiners in Optometry.

4.21   _____. PROCEEDINGS OF THE INTERNATIONAL CONFERENCE ON WOMEN IN HEALTH, JUNE 16-18, 1975, WASHINGTON, D.C. DHEW publication no. (HRA) 76-51. Health Manpower References. Washington, D.C.: Government Printing Office, 1976.

Covers current status of women as health care providers in the United States and other selected countries; approaches to correct the underrepresentation of women; improving the utilization of women already in the health professions; organization of nurses and allied health workers; and role of women in decision making. Includes many charts and tables.

Health Resources

4.22 _____. SUPPLY, NEED, AND DISTRIBUTION OF ANESTHESIOLOGISTS AND NURSE ANESTHETISTS IN THE U.S., 1972 AND 1980. By Pamela C. Roddy and Robert Hambleton. Washington, D.C.: Government Printing Office, 1977.

> Analysis of supply of M.D. anesthetists, nurse anesthetists, and estimation of need and supply for 1980 by state. Shows active practitioners, population to practitioner ratio, and shortage or surplus for 1972.

4.23 _____. THE SUPPLY OF HEALTH MANPOWER: 1970 PROFILES AND PROJECTIONS TO 1990. DHEW publication no. (HRA) 75-38 or NTIS PB-239 947/AS. Washington, D.C.: Government Printing Office, 1974.

> Presents comprehensive current and future profiles of health manpower supply. Detailed statistical and analytical material on the current profile and projected supply for: physicians, medical specialists, veterinarians, registered nurses, dentists, optometrists, pharmacists, podiatrists, and allied health occupations. Approximately 125 statistical tables.

4.24 _____. SURVEY OF SELECTED HOSPITAL MANPOWER, FEBRUARY 1973, PRELIMINARY REPORT. DHEW publication no. (HRA) 74-26. Washington, D.C.: Government Printing Office, 1974.

> Provides estimates of the numbers employed and the numbers of positions vacant for fourteen allied health occupations in community hospitals for the United States, four regions, and nine geographic divisions.

4.25 _____. WOMEN IN HEALTH CAREERS. DHEW publication no. (HRA) 76-55. Washington, D.C.: Government Printing Office, 1976.

> Covers women in the United States and other selected countries with emphasis on the United States. Contains information by sex for medical practitioners, education and enrollments, and specialization.

4.26 U.S. Bureau of Health Manpower. Division of Manpower Analysis. REPORT TO THE CONGRESS ON THE STATUS OF HEALTH PROFESSIONS PERSONNEL IN THE UNITED STATES. DHEW publication no. (HRA) 78-93. Hyattsville, Md.: 1978.

> An extensive report with numerous tables. Devotes a chapter to each major health profession. Projections to 1990.

Health Resources

4.27 U.S. Bureau of Health Manpower. Division of Nursing. NURSING PERSONNEL IN HOSPITALS: 1970 SURVEY OF HOSPITALS REGISTERED WITH THE AMERICAN HOSPITAL ASSOCIATION. DHEW publication no. (HRA) 75-16. Health Manpower References. Washington, D.C.: Government Printing Office, 1975.

> Presents data for nursing personnel employed in hospitals registered with the AHA. Projects data on the number of nursing personnel employed in these hospitals during the period 1-7 November 1970. Shows the number of nurses in a particular personnel category by type and ownership of hospital in each table as well as distribution of nursing personnel in hospitals by type, ownership, size and geographic location of the hospital.

4.28 _____. NURSING PERSONNEL IN HOSPITALS: 1972 PUBLIC HEALTH SURVEY. DHEW publication no. (HRA) 75-33 or NTIS PB 239-745. Health Manpower References. Springfield, Va.: National Technical Information Service, 1974.

> Presents data for nursing personnel employed in hospitals not registered with AHA. Projects data on the number of nursing personnel employed in these hospitals during the period 5-11 November 1972. Also shows the number of nurses in a particular personnel category by type and ownership of hospital. Gives summary tables which show distribution of nursing personnel in hospitals by type, ownership, size, and geographic location of the hospital.

4.29 _____. SURVEY OF FOREIGN NURSE GRADUATES. DHEW publication no. (HRA) 76-13. Health Manpower References. Washington, D.C.: Government Printing Office, 1976.

> Conducted by the American Nurses Association and supported by a Division of Nursing grant. Presents data on FNG's by state, countries of nursing education, number of FNG's taking and passing the State Board Test Pool Examination (SBTPE), those obtaining temporary permits to practice, marital status, type of nursing education, year of graduation, nursing experience, and educational differences.

4.30 _____. SURVEY OF REGISTERED NURSES EMPLOYED IN PHYSICIANS OFFICES, SEPTEMBER 1973. DHEW publication no. (HRA) 75-50. Health Manpower References. Washington, D.C.: Government Printing Office, 1975.

> Survey presents tables on the characteristics of nurses, employment conditions (income and benefits), activities performed, and participation in continuing education.

Health Resources

4.31 U.S. Bureau of Health Resources Development. CHARACTERISTICS OF BLACK PHYSICIANS IN THE U.S.: FINDINGS FROM A SURVEY. BHRD 75-147. Washington, D.C.: 1975.

Report on demographic and professional characteristics of black physicians in 1972. Tables present data by age, sex, medical school of graduation, and specialty.

4.32 _____. NURSING PERSONNEL IN HOSPITALS REGISTERED WITH AHA. DHEW publication no. (HRA) 75-16. Washington, D.C.: Government Printing Office, 1975.

Presents in tabular form information on staffing patterns on nearly sixty categories of hospital personnel. Primarily intended as a sourcebook on nursing manpower in AHA registered hospitals.

4.33 U.S. Division of Health Manpower Intelligence. REGISTERED PHARMACISTS IN (STATE), 1973. Washington, D.C.: 1973.

Separate reports for each state in the United States, the District of Columbia, and Puerto Rico. Manpower statistics by the following variables: age, sex, years of education, county, principal place of practice, and hours worked per week for 1973 in each report.

4.34 U.S. Health Resources Administration. STUDY OF PARTICIPATION OF WOMEN IN THE HEALTH CARE INDUSTRY LABOR FORCE. 4 vols. DHEW publication no. (HRA) 77-644. Washington, D.C.: Government Printing Office, 1977.

Report consists of the following volumes: (1) EXECUTIVE SUMMARY; (2) ANALYSIS OF WOMEN IN THE HEALTH LABOR FORCE; (3) Appendix A, HISTORICAL REVIEW OF WOMEN IN DENTISTRY: AN ANNOTATED BIBLIOGRAPHY; (4) Appendix B, MATERIALS RELATED TO THE STUDY OF WOMEN IN THE HEALTH LABOR FORCE. Gives data on demographic characteristics, perceptions of family and social attitudes, education, work experience and household arrangements. Covers licensed practical nurses (LPNs), registered nurses (RNs), dental hygienists, dentists, and health care administrators.

4.35 U.S. National Center for Health Statistics. DATA ON HEALTH RESOURCES: MANPOWER AND FACILITIES. Vital and Health Statistics Series, no. 14. Washington, D.C.: Government Printing Office, 1963-- . Irregular.

(See no. 4.4.)

Health Resources

4.36 _____. DECENNIAL CENSUS DATA FOR SELECTED HEALTH OCCUPATIONS: UNITED STATES, 1970. DHEW publication no. (HRA) 76-1231. Washington, D.C.: Government Printing Office, 1975.

This report considers the following demographic characteristics of twenty-eight categories of health practitioners: sex, ethnic composition, patterns of residence, and ratio per 100,000 resident population. Includes data for the nation, for states, and for eighty-three SMSA's having a population of 250,000 or more as of April 1, 1970.

4.37 _____. HEALTH MANPOWER. A COUNTY AND METROPOLITAN AREA DATA BOOK, 1972-75. DHEW publication no. (HRA) 76-1234. Washington, D.C.: Government Printing Office, 1976.

Provides counts of professional persons employed in nine health occupations in the nation's counties and metropolitan areas. Covers the following nine types of professionals: (1) dentists; (2) registered occupational therapists; (3) optometrists; (4) physicians, doctors of medicine; (5) physicians, doctors of osteopathy; (6) psychiatrists; (7) registered nurses; (8) pharmacists; (9) veterinarians.

4.38 _____. HEALTH RESOURCES STATISTICS: HEALTH MANPOWER AND FACILITIES. Washington, D.C.: Government Printing Office, 1965-- . Annual.

(See no. 4.5.)

4.39 U.S. National Institute of Neurological and Communicative Disorders and Stroke. NINCDS MANPOWER SURVEYS. Washington, D.C.: Government Printing Office, 1977.

Series of five reports prepared by nongovernment organizations under contract which present data and analysis for making projections to 1985 and concern disciplines relevant to the institute. Contains statistical detail concerning demographic characteristics and training, professional activities, demand for services and manpower needs, utilization of hospitals, incidence and prevalence of treated diseases, and conditions. Reports titled as follows: (1) NEUROLOGICAL MANPOWER: A SURVEY, NINCDS Monograph no. 16; (2) SPEECH PATHOLOGY AND AUDIOLOGY: MANPOWER RESOURCES AND NEEDS, NINCDS Monograph no. 17; (3) OTORHINOLARYNGOLOGY: MANPOWER RESOURCES AND NEEDS, NINCDS Monograph no. 18; (4) NEUROSURGERY MANPOWER: A SURVEY, NINCDS. Monograph no. 19; (5) MANPOWER IN BASIC NEUROLOGIC AND COMMUNICATIVE SCIENCES: A SURVEY, NINCDS Monograph no. 20.

Health Resources

4.40   Urban and Rural Systems Associates. EXPLORATORY STUDY OF WOMEN IN THE HEALTH PROFESSIONS SCHOOLS. 11 vols. Washington, D.C.: Women's Action Program, DHEW, 1976.

>   Focuses on eight health professions: medicine, osteopathic medicine, dentistry, veterinary medicine, optometry, podiatry, pharmacy, and public health. Covers only Caucasian women and not minority women. Presents data analysis, findings, conclusions, and recommendations, with statistical tables in the appendixes in volume 1. Covers the individual professions including statistical information throughout each report in volumes 2 through 9. Contains an annotated bibliography on the subject in volume 10 and the EXECUTIVE SUMMARY in volume 11.

HEALTH EDUCATION

Sources of data for health professions education have been included in this chapter because those being educated are potentially part of the nation's health manpower resources.

Data concerning education in the health professions come largely from the professional associations, the American Association of Medical Colleges, the U.S. Bureau of Health Manpower, and the U.S. National Center for Health Statistics.

The following publications cover data about medical schools, faculty and students. One may note that they reflect to some degree the current concern over the participation of women and minorities in the health professions.

4.41   American Dental Association. ANNUAL REPORT ON DENTAL EDUCATION. Chicago: 1967-68-- .

>   Contains information on dental schools, admissions, enrollment (by sex), graduates (sex and state), student educational expenses, and faculty positions. Additional information, such as auxilliary dental education in supplements.

4.42   American Medical Association. MEDICAL EDUCATION IN THE UNITED STATES. ANNUAL REPORT. Chicago: 1901-- .

>   First published in 1901 in the JOURNAL OF THE AMERICAN MEDICAL ASSOCIATION and now a separate issue. Currently presents information in seven sections, some narrative and some statistical: Section 1, financial information; Section 2, student enrollment, faculty, and curriculum; Section 3, graduate medical education; Section 4, continuing medical education; Section 5, allied medical education; Section 6, programs sponsored by government agencies; Section 7, public health education.

Health Resources

4.43 Association of American Medical Colleges. Office of Minority Affairs. MINORITY STUDENT OPPORTUNITIES IN UNITED STATES MEDICAL SCHOOLS, 1975-76. Washington, D.C.: 1975.

Designed as a source of information for prospective minority medical students and their advisors. Provides minority application and enrollment statistics for 108 of the 114 medical schools in the United States. Includes statistics on number of minority students who applied, number accepted for admission, number who matriculated, and total number of minority students.

4.44 Commission on Physicians for the Future. PHYSICIANS FOR THE FUTURE. New York: Josiah Macy, Jr. Foundation, 1976.

An analysis of the demand for physicians and the ability of the educational system to respond to it. Statistical background for the report and many tables on both the supply of physicians and enrollments in medical schools in the appendix. Includes data on foreign medical graduates. Extensive bibliography and list of sources for all statistics cited.

4.45 Larson, Thomas A., and Farlee, Coralie. NATIONAL ESTIMATES OF FACULTY MANPOWER IN U.S. MEDICAL SCHOOLS, FINAL REPORT. Washington, D.C.: Association of American Medical Colleges, 1977.

Data from three sources: the AAMC-AMA Liaison Committee on Medical Education, the annual AAMC Salary, and the AAMC Faculty Roster System. Faculty counts by rank and degree, department, or specialty in each annual report, 1970-75. Also national estimates of annual faculty appointment, turnover, and promotion.

4.46 National League for Nursing. SOME STATISTICS ON BACCALAUREATE AND HIGHER DEGREE PROGRAMS IN NURSING-1975-76. Publication no. 19-1649. New York: 1977.

Supplements data published annually in NURSING OUTLOOK and statistical summaries published in the 1976 edition of STATE-APPROVED SCHOOLS OF NURSING. Gives statistics for enrollments and graduations of nurses in doctoral, masters, and baccalaureate programs. Totals for 1965-75. Also covers financial assistance statistics. Breaks down by geographic region and functional area of study.

4.47 U.S. Bureau of Health Manpower. HEALTH PROFESSIONS SCHOOLS: SELECTED ENROLLMENT DATA. Health Manpower References. Washington, D.C.: Government Printing Office, 1965/76-- . Annual.

Health Resources

Annual report which provides enrollment data in individual health professions schools assisted by the U.S. Bureau of Health Manpower. Shows data by enrollment for each year of study, total enrollment and graduates for each academic year. Also shows data for each discipline by school listed alphabetically by state. Disciplines include medicine, osteopathy, dentistry, physician's assistants, dental therapy, optometry, pharmacy, podiatry, and veterinary medicine.

4.48 _____. INSTITUTIONAL CHARACTERISTICS OF U.S. MEDICAL SCHOOLS, 1975-1976, FINAL REPORT. DHEW publication no. (HRA) 78-79. Health Manpower References. Washington, D.C.: Government Printing Office, 1978.

Describes medical schools in the United States in terms of their curricula, students, faculty, finances, teaching hospitals, and clinics. Includes over one hundred tables. Latest data available in 1977.

4.49 "U.S. Medical Student Enrollment 1972-73 through 1976-77." JOURNAL OF MEDICAL EDUCATION 52 (February 1977): 164-66.

In the datagram section of the journal. Presents information about first-year U.S. medical school enrollments by sex, minority group, and foreign student variables. Also presents information for total U.S. medical school enrollments by the same variables. Similar subjects covered in other datagram sections.

4.50 U.S. National Center for Education Statistics. ANALYSIS OF DOCTOR'S DEGREES AWARDED TO MEN AND WOMEN 1970-71 THROUGH 1974-75. By Mary D. Ott. DHEW publication no. (NCES) 77-333. Washington, D.C.: 1977.

Report on the number of doctoral degree recipients by sex, subject area, detailed field of study, institutional control, region, and state.

4.51 _____. WOMEN'S PARTICIPATION IN FIRST-PROFESSIONAL DEGREE PROGRAMS IN MEDICINE, DENTISTRY, VETERINARY MEDICINE, AND LAW, 1969-70 THROUGH 1974-75. DHEW publication no. (NCES) 76-023. Washington, D.C.: Government Printing Office, 1976.

Report on the number of women enrolled and receiving degrees in first professional degree programs in four disciplines, school years 1969-70 to 1974-75. Data are from NCES surveys and professional associations.

Chapter 5
HEALTH SERVICES UTILIZATION

There is a multiplicity of sources both public and private for data on health services utilization, but there is a paucity of data. Serious gaps in utilization data include services provided by nursing homes, extended care facilities, and all ambulatory care facilities.

The most notable publications from private organizations are HOSPITAL STATISTICS (see no. 5.2) and LENGTH OF STAY IN PAS HOSPITALS (see no. 5.5). An excellent study of the utilization of surgical services can be found in SURGERY IN THE UNITED STATES (see no. 1.103). The U.S. National Center for Health Statistics Series 13, DATA ON HEALTH RESOURCES UTILIZATION (see no. 5.13), provides data from a national sample survey on the utilization of various facilities. Data related to Medicare and Medicaid utilization are now collected by the Health Care Financing Administration. This responsibility formerly rested with the Social Security Administration. However, at this time information about which publications from the U.S. Social Security Administration will be continued by the Health Care Financing Administration is not available.

5.1   Alan Guttmacher Institute. CONTRACEPTIVE SERVICES FOR ADOLESCENTS: UNITED STATES, EACH STATE, AND COUNTY, 1975. New York: 1978.

   Presents a summary for the United States, each region, state, and county of the number of women aged fifteen to nineteen who are at risk of unintended pregnancy. Detailed tables of data on the number served and not served by clinic programs, and the percent distribution of patients served by agency type for each state and county, 1975.

5.2   American Hospital Association. HOSPITAL STATISTICS. Chicago: 1972-- . Annual.

   Previously part of the annual GUIDE ISSUE OF HOSPITALS. Issued separately since 1972. Series of tables covering, by various parameters, utilization, finance, personnel, facilities, and services. Updates of many of these tables published in

Health Services Utilization

the bimonthly issue of HOSPITALS dated the sixteenth of each month under the title "Hospital Indicators."

5.3   American Medical Association. REFERENCE DATA ON THE PROFILE OF MEDICAL PRACTICE. Chicago: 1971-- . Annual.

(See no. 1.94.)

5.4   Anderson, Ronald, et al. HEALTH SERVICE USE--NATIONAL TRENDS AND VARIATIONS, 1953-1971. DHEW publication no. (HSM) 73-3004. Rockville, Md.: 1973.

Report of survey findings on the use of health services. Tabulates regular source of care, physician care, hospital care, surgical procedures, obstetrical care, dental care, Medicaid utilization by state, disability days, and physician contacts. Presents information by such variables as age, race, income, residence, and year.

5.5   Commission on Professional and Hospital Activities. LENGTH OF STAY IN PAS HOSPITALS, BY DIAGNOSIS. Ann Arbor, Mich.: 1975-- .

Continues LENGTH OF STAY IN PAS HOSPITALS, UNITED STATES, 1969-74. Compiles data from individual patient discharge abstracts submitted by hospitals participating in the Professional Activity Study (PAS) of the Commission on Professional and Hospital Activities (CPHA). Shows stay distributions for patients discharged during 1975 from short-term nonfederal hospitals (2,117 hospitals) in length of stay tables. Makes distinctions between the stay for patients who were operated on as opposed to those who were not. Does not include patients who died, were transferred, or left against medical advice. Other books on length of stay by the CPHA: LENGTH OF STAY IN PAS HOSPITALS, BY DIAGNOSES, UNITED STATES, SOUTHERN REGION, 1975-- ; LENGTH OF STAY IN PAS HOSPITALS, BY DIAGNOSIS, UNITED STATES, NORTH CENTRAL REGION, 1975-- ; LENGTH OF STAY IN PAS HOSPITALS, BY DIAGNOSIS, UNITED STATES, NORTH EASTERN REGION, 1975-- ; LENGTH OF STAY IN PAS HOSPITALS, BY DIAGNOSIS, UNITED STATES, WESTERN REGION, 1975-- ; LENGTH OF STAY IN PAS HOSPITALS, BY DIAGNOSIS, CANADA, 1975-- .

5.5a   NATIONAL PRESCRIPTION AUDIT, COMPANY REPORT. TEN-YEAR TREND. Ambler, Pa.: IMS America, 1958-67-- . Annual.

Data from the National Prescription Audit presented by company name and number of different products appearing over the ten-year period. Gives total new prescriptions for company as well as total new prescription dollars at the manufacturers' level.

Health Services Utilization

5.5b NATIONAL PRESCRIPTION AUDIT, NATIONAL HOSPITAL SURVEY. GENERAL INFORMATION REPORT. 5 vols. Dedham, Mass.: R.A. Gosselin, 1966-71.

> Formerly: NATIONAL PRESCRIPTION AUDIT. GENERAL INFORMATION REPORT. Presents data about the hospital drug market. Shows leading ten therapeutic classes in order of dollar purchases by hospitals; leading two hundred products purchased, ranked by percent of drug purchases to hospitals; leading companies ranked by percent of drug purchases by hospitals.

5.5c NATIONAL PRESCRIPTION AUDIT, THERAPEUTIC CATEGORY REPORT. TEN YEAR TREND. Ambler, Pa.: IMS America, 1955-64-- . Annual.

> Established in 1952. Measures the rate at which drugs are sold to consumers. Data shows total new prescriptions, total new prescription dollars at the manufacturers' level, total new and refilled prescriptions, and percent of the market for each therapeutic category. Taken from a sample of pharmacy files audited for a number of days each month.

5.6 Newman, John F., and Anderson, Odin W. PATTERNS OF DENTAL SERVICES UTILIZATION IN THE UNITED STATES: A NATIONWIDE SOCIAL SURVEY. Research Services--Center for Health Administration Studies, no. 30. Chicago: University of Chicago, Center for Health Administration Studies, 1972.

> Data from a national sample of households which reflect overall population characteristics (age, sex, race, and income). Includes trends in utilization of services, social and economic variables in the use of services, utilization by type of service (cleaning, filling), effect of symptoms on utilization in conjunction with demographic and socioeconomic variables, and continuity of utilization.

5.7 Piore, Nora. A STATISTICAL PROFILE OF HOSPITAL OUTPATIENT SERVICES IN THE U.S.: PRESENT SCOPE AND POTENTIAL ROLE. New York: Association for Aid to Crippled Children, 1971.

> Provides an overview of the scope and characteristics of hospital based ambulatory care. Describes data presently available and data needed for analysis. Also sets forth some public policies which would lead to the use of hospital clinics and emergency rooms as a network of comprehensive health care centers.

5.8 Scitovsky, Anne A., and Snyder, Nelda M. MEDICAL CARE USE BY A GROUP OF FULLY INSURED AGED: A CASE STUDY. DHEW publication no. (HRA) 76-3129. Washington, D.C.: Government Printing Office, 1976.

Health Services Utilization

Examines the use of medical care by five hundred persons aged sixty-five and over, all of whom have a middle-to upper-middle-class background and access to medical services. Indicates the demand for medical services that older people might make if they had middle-class standards of medical care and services were provided free of charge. Gives utilization data for physician's services, hospital care, nursing home care, and other medical care services. Compares expenditures to the national average. Brief bibliography.

5.9 U.S. Bureau of Radiological Health. POPULATION EXPOSURE TO X-RAYS, U.S. 1970. DHEW publication no. (FDA) 73-8047. Washington, D.C.: Government Printing Office, 1973.

Provides estimates of population exposure by type of examination or procedure, and for various demographic and socioeconomic characteristics. Also presents data on types of facilities and specialties of persons administering the procedures. No data on the genetic or organ dose estimates for the population.

5.10 U.S. Center for Disease Control. ABORTION SURVEILLANCE. Atlanta, Ga.: 1972-- . Irregular.

Former title: FAMILY PLANNING EVALUATION: LEGAL ABORTIONS. Report on legal abortions reported by state health departments and hospitals in twenty-four states. Data by age, race, marital status, type of procedures, and weeks of gestation.

5.11 _____. UNITED STATES IMMUNIZATION SURVEY. Atlanta, Ga.: 1965-- . Annual.

Annual report on immunization data for poliomyelitis, diptheria-tetanus-pertussis, measles, rubella, mumps, influenza, and smallpox. Variables by age group, race, urban or rural, SMSA cities and others, and region. Estimates of data based on current population surveys done annually in September by the Census Bureau.

5.12 U.S. Indian Health Service. Office of Program Statistics. DISCHARGE SUMMARY. Rockville, Md.: 1957-- . Annual.

Summarizes inpatient data gathered from Indian Health Service Hospitals and other hospitals under contract. Focuses on trends in morbidity by age group, average length of stay, and sex. Gives special attention to high utilization rates for injuries and mental disorders.

Health Services Utilization

5.13   U.S. National Center for Health Statistics. DATA ON HEALTH RESOURCES UTILIZATION. Vital and Health Statistics Series, no. 13. Washington, D.C.: Government Printing Office, 1963-- . Irregular.

Offers statistics on the utilization of health manpower and facilities providing long-term care, ambulatory care, hospital care, and family planning services.

5.14   _____. NATIONAL REPORTING SYSTEM FOR FAMILY PLANNING SERVICES. Washington, D.C.: Government Printing Office, 1976-- . Annual.

Data on number and characteristics of persons receiving family planning services in public and private clinics.

5.15   _____. THE NATION'S USE OF HEALTH RESOURCES. DHEW publication no. (HRA) 77-1240. Washington, D.C.: Government Printing Office, 1977.

A compendium of the utilization of health resources. Includes a description and analysis by demographic characteristics of the users of health resources.

5.16   _____. STATE ESTIMATES OF DISABILITY AND UTILIZATION OF MEDICAL SERVICES: UNITED STATES, 1969-71. DHEW publication no. (HRA) 77-1241. Washington, D.C.: Government Printing Office, 1977.

Data from the NCHS Health Interview Survey. "Synthetic" estimates because they were not directly derived from survey results and the results are biased estimates. Presents tabular data by geographic (region and state) and socioeconomic variables. Is "in response to the continually growing demand for small area statistics on health-related topics."

5.17   U.S. National Institute of Mental Health. MENTAL HEALTH FACILITIES REPORTS. REPORT SERIES ON MENTAL HEALTH STATISTICS, SERIES A. Washington, D.C.: Government Printing Office, 1969-- . Irregular.

(See no. 3.41.)

5.18   U.S. Social Security Administration. Office of Research and Statistics. HEALTH INSURANCE FOR THE AGED: ANNUAL PROGRAM DATA. Washington, D.C.: 196?-- . Irregular.

The official statistical record of the Medicare program compiled and analyzed for each year. Designed to cover all areas of the Medicare program. Includes: Section 1, "Summary," capsulizes data for the hospital insurance and supplementary medical insurance program for the year. Also presents compara-

Health Services Utilization

tive data with previous years. 1.1, "Reimbursement by State and County," data published for 1969, 1970, 1971, 1972, and 1974–75. 1.2, "Utilization and Reimbursement by Person," data published for 1966, 1967, 1968, and 1969. 1.3, "Reimbursement--Geographic Index," data published for 1969, 1970, 1971, 1972, and 1973. Section 2, "Enrollment," contains Medicare enrollment data by age, race, sex, region, division, state of residence, and standard metropolitan statistical area. Data published for 1969, 1970, 1971, and 1972–74. Section 3, "Participating Providers," presents data on such providers of service under Medicare as hospitals, home health agencies, independent laboratories, and skilled nursing facilities. Data published for 1969, 1970, 1971, and 1972–74. Section 4, "Inpatient Care," 4.1, "Short-Stay Hospital Utilization," presents utilization data for inpatient care for short-stay hospitals. Data published for 1966, 1967, and 1968–72.

5.19 _____. HEALTH INSURANCE NOTES. Washington, D.C.: 1965-- . Irregular.

Continuing series of reports on the structure and utilization of Medicare hospital insurance programs. Includes members, eligibility, and characteristics of enrollees. Issued on a more or less monthly basis.

5.20 _____. LENGTH OF STAY BY DIAGNOSIS. Washington, D.C.: 1969-- . Irregular.

National and regional data on the number of Medicare discharges from short-stay hospitals, the mean and median length of stay, and percentile distribution of days of care for selected diagnoses. Gives data on patient age, presence of secondary or complicating conditions, and whether or not surgery was performed for each diagnosis. Data published for 1969, 1970, and 1971.

Chapter 6
HEALTH CARE COSTS AND EXPENDITURES

Data on health care costs and expenditures are again somewhat scattered among public and private sources. The references listed in this chapter represent the best of what is available including journal articles which are updated regularly (see no. 6.11). The publications include data on insurance costs (public and private), fees, national and personal health care expenditures, and costs of treatment and hospitalization for certain illnesses. The area with the most inadequate data is that concerning the direct and indirect costs of specific illnesses. These data may sometimes be found in journal articles in which studies are reported.

6.1 American Council of Life Insurance. LIFE INSURANCE FACT BOOK. New York: 1946-- . Annual.

    A statistical portrait of the life insurance business. Includes information about health insurance benefit payments provided by life insurance companies.

6.2 American Dental Association. 1975 FEE SURVEY. Chicago: 1976.

    Data on fees from a total of 6,400 dentists. Lists types of dental services by general practitioners and selected specialists. Only national data.

6.3 _____. 1977 SURVEY OF DENTAL PRACTICE. Chicago: 1979.

    Covers 1976 data of average net and average gross income of independent dentists by state. Includes data on number of patients seen per week.

6.4 American Medical Association. REFERENCE DATA ON SOCIOECONOMIC ISSUES OF HEALTH. Chicago: 1971-- . Annual.

    (See no. 1.99.)

Health Care Costs and Expenditures

6.5 _____. REFERENCE DATA ON THE PROFILE OF MEDICAL PRACTICE. Chicago: 1971-- . Annual.

(See no. 1.94.)

6.6 Berry, Ralph E. THE ECONOMIC COST OF ALCOHOL ABUSE. New York: Free Press, 1977.

Includes statistics on the cost of lost production, health care costs, cost of motor vehicle accidents, cost of fires, cost of crime and the cost of "social responses" such as rehabilitation, public assistance, workman's compensation, fire protection, and criminal justice.

6.7 Cooper, Barbara S. COMPENDIUM OF NATIONAL HEALTH EXPENDITURES DATA. DHEW publication no. (SSA) 76-11927. Washington, D.C.: Government Printing Office, 1977.

Collection of all available data on health expenditures. Makes no attempt at analysis. Presents statistics on trends in health expenditures, 1929-74; total national health expenditures; expenditures under public programs; private health insurance; and expenditures by age groups. Lists sources.

6.8 Cooper, Barbara S., and Rice, Dorothy P. "The Economic Cost of Illness Revisited." SOCIAL SECURITY BULLETIN 39, no. 2 (1976): 21-36.

Updates the earlier study by Dorothy P. Rice of the cost of illness (see no. 6.17). Presents costs in terms of the direct costs for prevention, detection and treatment, and the indirect costs due to disability and premature death for the sixteen major diagnostic categories of illnesses. Covers general categories of disease, although there is a discussion of the cost of stroke which is not covered in the tables. Diagnostic categories are infective and parasitic diseases; neoplasms; endocrine, nutritional, and metabolic diseases; diseases of the blood and blood-forming organs; mental disorders; diseases of the nervous system and sense organs; diseases of the circulatory system; diseases of the respiratory system; diseases of the digestive system, diseases of the genitourinary system; complications of pregnancy, childbirth, and the puerperium; diseases of the skin and subcutaneous tissue; diseases of the musculoskeletal system and connective tissue; congenital anomalies; and accidents, poisonings, and violence.

6.9 Cooper, Barbara S., and Worthington, Nancy L. PERSONAL HEALTH CARE EXPENDITURES BY STATE. 2 vols. DHEW publication no. (SSA) 73-11906. Washington, D.C.: Government Printing Office, 1973.

Health Care Costs and Expenditures

Volume 1, PUBLIC FUNDS, 1966 AND 1969, presents personal health care expenditures under public programs. Gives state data for each public program by source of funds and by type of expenditure. Volume 2, PUBLIC AND PRIVATE FUNDS, 1966 AND 1969, presents state estimates of total spending by source of funds and type of expenditure.

6.10 Gibson, Robert M., and Fisher, Charles R. "National Health Expenditures, Fiscal Year 1977." SOCIAL SECURITY BULLETIN 40, no. 7 (1978): 3-20.

An annual article which presents information for the past fiscal year. Includes statistics on aggregate and per capita national health expenditures; type of expenditures and source of funds; personal health care expenditures by type of expenditure; expenditures for health services by public program and source of funds; trends for 1929-77.

6.11 Health Insurance Institute. SOURCEBOOK OF HEALTH INSURANCE DATA. New York: 1959-- . Annual.

Provides the latest available data for the year published on the major forms of health insurance as well as medical care costs. Data on medical care costs include: personal and national expenditures, consumer price index, and hospital charges and costs. Also some data on morbidity trends.

6.12 Hu, Teh-wei, ed. INTERNATIONAL HEALTH COSTS AND EXPENDITURES. DHEW publication no. (NIH) 76-1067. Geographic Health Studies. John E. Fogarty International Center for Advanced Study in the Health Sciences. Washington, D.C.: Government Printing Office, 1976.

Proceedings of a conference in health economics covering papers discussing health costs in Belgium, Canada, Denmark, France, the Netherlands, Romania, Sweden, the United Kingdom, the United States, and West Germany. Many tables and charts with data on health expenditures in each paper. Makes comparisons between the United States and other countries as well.

6.13 Institute of Medicine. COSTS OF EDUCATION IN THE HEALTH PROFESSIONS: REPORT OF A STUDY, PARTS I AND II. Washington, D.C.: National Academy of Sciences, 1974.

A study which determines the costs of education in the eight health fields: medicine, osteopathy, dentistry, optometry, pharmacy, podiatry, veterinary medicine, and nursing. Contains data on the health professional schools, the cost of education and variations in each of the eight fields in part 2. Includes a total of 161 tables.

Health Care Costs and Expenditures

6.14   Koleda, Michael. THE FEDERAL HEALTH DOLLAR. Washington, D.C.: Center for Health Policy Studies, National Planning Association, 1977.

   Provides an overview of the expenditures of the federal government for health-related activities for 1969-76. Includes health research, health manpower training, provision of health services, construction of health facilities, prevention and control of health problems, and improving the delivery of health care. Makes no attempt at evaluation.

6.14a   LILLY DIGEST. Indianapolis, Ind.: Eli Lilly and Co., 1932-- . Annual.

   An annual compilation of financial information submitted voluntarily by independent community pharmacists in the United States. Includes operating cost figures, total sales, and daily prescription activity. Gives no figures for specific drugs or drug classes. Meant to be a reflection of pharmacy operating figures and be a guide for pharmacy managements.

6.15   Marquis, Kent, et al. THE MEASUREMENT OF EXPENDITURES FOR OUTPATIENT PHYSICIAN AND DENTAL SERVICES: METHODOLOGICAL FINDINGS FROM THE HEALTH INSURANCE STUDY. Santa Monica, Calif.: Rand, 1976.

   Examines survey techniques that can be used to obtain data on health expenditures for outpatient physician and dental services.

6.16   Pharmaceutical Manufacturers Association. PRESCRIPTION DRUG INDUSTRY FACTBOOK. Washington, D.C.: 1965-- . Annual.

   A reference guide concerning social and economic aspects of prescription pharmaceutical manufacture and distribution. Contains statistics on pharmaceutical prices such as average prescription costs, drugstore prescription sales, and wholesale price index by therapeutic class. Also data on consumer expenditures for prescription pharmaceuticals and other national health care expenditure data.

6.17   Rice, Dorothy P. ESTIMATING THE COST OF ILLNESS. Health Economics Series, no. 6. U.S. Public Health Service, publication no. 947-6. Washington, D.C.: Government Printing Office, 1966.

   Presents a framework for calculating the economic costs of illness, disability and death and performs the calculations. Discusses the problems involved in measuring annual direct costs of illness, describes the procedures adopted, and presents data for selected types of health expenditures in 1963

Health Care Costs and Expenditures

by diagnosis in part 1. Deals with the annual indirect losses associated with illness, disability and death in part 2. Includes the economic concepts, estimating procedures and estimates of the total man-years lost, and productivity losses resulting from morbidity and mortality in 1963 for each diagnostic category. Presents the methodology and resulting estimates of the present value of the future earnings for those people who died in 1963 in part 3.

6.18 Rufener, Brent L., et al. MANAGEMENT EFFECTIVENESS MEASURES FOR NIDA DRUG ABUSE TREATMENT PROGRAMS, FINAL REPORT. 2 vols. Rockville, Md.: National Institute on Drug Abuse, 1976.

Report on cost-benefit for five drug abuse treatment modalities: methadone maintenance, therapeutic community, outpatient drug free, outpatient detoxification, and inpatient detoxification. Published in two volumes: volume 1, COST BENEFIT ANALYSIS and volume 2, COST TO SOCIETY OF DRUG ABUSE.

6.19 Scitovsky, Anne A., and McCall, Nelda. CHANGES IN THE COSTS OF TREATMENT OF SELECTED ILLNESSES, 1951-1964-1971. DHEW publication no. (HRA) 77-3161. NCHSR Research Digest Series. Rockville, Md.: Health Resources Administration, 1976.

A study to determine what light the data would shed on the U.S. Bureau of Labor Statistics medical care price index for the period 1964-71 and to analyze the effects of changes in treatment on costs. Shows average costs for selected illnesses and the percentage change in average cost 1951-64 and 1964-71 in tables. Details the number of diagnostic and other services per care; and the average number of physician visits and average length of hospital stay per case, 1951, 1964 and 1971. Examines otitis media in children, acute appendicitis, maternity, breast cancer, forearm fractures in children, pneumonia, duodenal ulcer, and myocardial infarction.

6.20 U.S. Congress. Congressional Budget Office. LONG-TERM CARE: ACTUAL COST ESTIMATES. Washington, D.C.: Government Printing Office, 1977.

Presents detailed information on the demand for long-term health and social services, the existing supply of those services, and the cost for increasing them. Tables include sources and uses of funds; estimated spending fiscal years 1977-85; estimated effect on spending for home health services fiscal years 1979-85.

Health Care Costs and Expenditures

6.21 U.S. Council on Wage and Price Stability. A STUDY OF PHYSICIANS' FEES. By Zachary Y. Dyckman. Washington, D.C.: Government Printing Office, 1978.

> Discussion accompanied by charts and tables of trends in physicians' fees and expenditures for physicians' services. Includes trend data of fees relative to other occupations and variations of fee levels across metropolitan areas. Data primarily taken from MEDICAL ECONOMICS surveys.

6.22 U.S. Health Services and Mental Health Administration. DETERMINANTS OF EXPENDITURES FOR PHYSICIANS' SERVICES IN THE UNITED STATES, 1948-1968. DHEW publication no. (HSM) 73-3013. Washington, D.C.: Government Printing Office, 1973.

> Examines expenditures for physician services over time, 1948-68; and across states, 1966. Breaks data down by such items as quantity of services, source of payment, per capita income, age, sex, and state.

6.23 U.S. National Cancer Institute. Biometry Branch. THIRD NATIONAL CANCER SURVEY: HOSPITALIZATIONS AND PAYMENTS TO HOSPITALS. PART A: SUMMARY. DHEW publication no. (NIH) 76-1094. Bethesda, Md.: 1976.

> Presents data from the first major study undertaken by the National Cancer Institute which directly measured hospitalizations for specific cancer patients. Correlates costs with a variety of factors including age at time of diagnosis, survival, site of cancer, extent of disease, medical procedure, admission sequence, and source and number of payers. Also provides a complete history of payments to hospitals for inpatient care over a two-year follow-up period.

6.24 U.S. National Institute of Neurological and Communicative Disorders and Stroke. NEUROLOGICAL AND COMMUNICATIVE DISORDERS: ESTIMATED NUMBERS AND COST. DHEW publication no. (NIH) 77-152. Washington, D.C.: Government Printing Office, 1976.

> Pamphlet that presents a table of neurological and sensory disorders, and the mortality, estimated total cases, and estimated annual cost of care. Obtained some estimated cases from voluntary organizations.

6.25 U.S. National Institutes of Health. Nephrology Cost Group. HEMODIALYSIS COSTS IN THE U.S. By Paul A. Hoffstein. PB 245-805. Springfield, Va.: National Technical Information Service, 1974.

Health Care Costs and Expenditures

Report on costs of performing chronic hemodialytic therapy in programs of five representative dialysis centers. Presents costs per treatment for personnel, supplies, equipment, and other direct or indirect costs.

6.26 U.S. Social Security Administration. Office of Research and Statistics. MEDICAL CARE COSTS AND PRICES: BACKGROUND BOOK. DHEW publication no. (SSA) 75-11909. Washington, D.C.: Government Printing Office, 1975.

Comprehensive data on the costs and prices of hospital care, physicians' and dentists' services, and on significant trends in these expenses.

6.27 _____. PRESCRIPTION DRUG DATA SUMMARY. Washington, D.C.: 1970-- . Annual.

Current and trend statistics on expenditures for drugs, numbers of drugs prescribed, prescription prices, and new drugs developed.

6.28 _____. RESEARCH AND STATISTICS NOTE. Washington, D.C.: 1965-- . Monthly.

Continuing series of reports on various aspects of social security programs. Includes health expenditures, hospital and medical care costs, veterans programs, and workman's compensation. Issued on a more or less monthly basis.

6.29 _____. SIZE AND SHAPE OF THE MEDICAL CARE DOLLAR: CHARTBOOK 1975. Washington, D.C.: Government Printing Office, 1976.

Facts about the medical dollar--who pays, what and how much is bought, and for whom it is spent. Shows trends in medical care outlays, the causes of rising hospital costs, and roles of private and public financing.

6.30 _____. SOCIAL SECURITY BULLETIN: ANNUAL STATISTICAL SUPPLEMENT. Washington, D.C.: Government Printing Office, 1956-- .

Annual report on social security funds, coverage, benefits, and beneficiaries. Presents detailed breakdown of OASDHI coverage and benefits by age, sex, and race. Also a summary of black lung and public assistance programs.

6.31 _____. STUDY OF PHYSICIANS' INCOME IN THE PRE-MEDICARE PERIOD, 1965. DHW publication no. (SSA) 76-11932. Washington, D.C.: Government Printing Office, 1976.

Presents income statistics for physicians by specialty and practice characteristics. Intended to provide pre-Medicare baseline data for assessing Medicare program impact on physician income.

Chapter 7
POPULATION CHARACTERISTICS

Vital and health statistics have no meaning unless they can be related to the population. In other words, the data which describe the population form the basis for analyzing health data. A population profile is essential to determine what the utilization, morbidity or mortality figures really mean. The population profile includes: (1) demographic characteristics such as age, race, and sex; (2) socioeconomic characteristics such as income, education, and occupation; and (3) housing characteristics.

Statistics on the U.S. population have been collected and published in decennial censuses since 1790 with increasing detail. Population data therefore are more complete and more detailed than health data (which was also collected during the decennial census until 1900!). The Census Bureau continues to have this responsibility and operates under the requirements of the Constitution of the United States.

Listed below are the major publications series of the Census Bureau. The DETAILED CHARACTERISTICS of the census of population (see no. 7.8) and the CURRENT POPULATION REPORTS, Series P-26 (see no. 7.2) are most useful for small area data.

7.1 U.S. Bureau of the Census, CONGRESSIONAL DISTRICT DATA BOOK. Washington, D.C.: Government Printing Office, 1973.

Contains population and housing data from the 1970 census broken down geographically by congressional district.

7.2 _____. COUNTY AND CITY DATA BOOK, 1977. Washington, D.C.: Government Printing Office, 1978.

Presents data from the most recent censuses and from other government agencies and private sources. Provides statistics for every county and for every city with a population of 25,000 or more, as well as for metropolitan areas, states, regions, and census divisions. Available on computer tape.

Population Characteristics

7.3 _____. CURRENT POPULATION REPORTS, FEDERAL-STATE COOPERATIVE PROGRAM FOR POPULATION ESTIMATES. Series P-26. Washington, D.C.: Government Printing Office, 1969-- . Irregular.

    Data for states, counties, SMSA's on the total population and components of change (births, deaths, and migration).

7.4 _____. CURRENT POPULATION REPORTS, POPULATION CHARACTERISTICS. Series P-20. Washington, D.C.: Government Printing Office, n.d. Irregular.

    Latest national data on specified characteristics of the population.

7.5 _____. CURRENT POPULATION REPORTS, POPULATION ESTIMATES AND PROJECTIONS: POPULATION ESTIMATES FOR COUNTIES, INCORPORATED PLACES AND SELECTED MINOR CIVIL DIVISIONS. Series P-25. Washington, D.C.: Government Printing Office, 1947-- . Irregular.

7.6 _____. A STATISTICAL PORTRAIT OF WOMEN IN THE UNITED STATES: CURRENT POPULATION REPORTS. SPECIAL STUDIES. Washington, D.C.: Government Printing Office, 1976.

    Presents a statistical portrait showing "the role of women in the United States during the 20th century." Takes data from government sources: surveys, decennial censuses, vital statistics, and administrative records. Provides selected data in a historical framework, beginning in 1950, or earlier if statistics are available. Traces trends among women in the areas of population growth and composition, longevity, mortality and health, residence and migration, marital and family status, fertility, education, labor force participation, occupation and industry, work experience, income and poverty status, voting and public office holding, and crime and victimization. Discusses comparisons of black and white women separately; includes recent data for women of Spanish origin.

7.7 _____. URBAN ATLAS: TRACT DATA FOR STANDARD METROPOLITAN STATISTICAL AREAS. Washington, D.C.: Government Printing Office, 1974.

    Series contains twelve large map charts for each of the sixty-five largest SMSA's in the United States and presents population characteristics, socioeconomic data, and housing characteristics.

7.8 _____. U.S. CENSUS OF POPULATION-1(5): DETAILED CHARACTERISTICS, FINAL REPORT. Series PC (1) D1--PC (1) D52. Washington, D.C.: Government Printing Office, 1970-72.

Population Characteristics

Data for states, cities, SMSA's by age, race, state or country of birth, parentage, residence, education, number of children, veteran status, place of work, occupation, and income.

7.9 _____. U.S. CENSUS OF POPULATION-1970: EMPLOYMENT PROFILES OF SELECTED LOW-INCOME AREAS, FINAL REPORT. Series PHC (3)1--PHC (3)76. Washington, D.C.: Government Printing Office, 1972.

Covers sixty urban areas and seven rural areas. Data on the labor force, employment status, occupation, and industry.

7.10 _____. U.S. CENSUS OF POPULATION, 1970: VOLUME II, SUBJECT REPORTS. FINAL REPORT. LOW-INCOME AREAS IN LARGE CITIES. Series PC (2)-9B. Washington, D.C.: Government Printing Office, 1973.

Covers sixty largest cities with data on selected demographic characteristics, socioeconomic, and housing characteristics with emphasis on income levels.

7.11 U.S. Department of Labor. Bureau of Labor Statistics. BLACK AMERICANS, A CHARTBOOK, BULLETIN 1699. Washington, D.C.: Government Printing Office, 1971.

Charts on migration and population, employment, income, poverty, family, vital statistics and health, housing, crime, and citizenship for black people are presented.

7.12 _____. HANDBOOK OF LABOR STATISTICS. Washington, D.C.: Government Printing Office, 1936-- . Annual.

Makes available in one volume the majority of data collected by BLS. Completes each table historically, beginning with the earliest reliable and consistent data. Groups data under economic subject headings.

7.13 _____. U.S. WORKING WOMAN: A DATABOOK. Bulletin 1977. Washington, D.C.: Government Printing Office, 1977.

Statistical report on the changing role of women in the labor force. Text with tables and charts on labor force participation of women. Includes information on employment, marital status, income, education, job tenure, work life expectancy, and other social and demographic characteristics.

7.14 U.S. National Criminal Justice Information and Statistics Service. SOURCEBOOK OF CRIMINAL JUSTICE STATISTICS. Washington, D.C.: Government Printing Office, 1974-- . Annual.

Population Characteristics

        Comprehensive compilations of statistics on criminal justice and related matters. Includes reported marihuana use among the general population by demographic characteristics among the adult and youth population. Also forcible rapes: characteristics of the victim and offender by sex, race, and age.

7.15   U.S. Social Security Administration. Office of Research and Statistics. EARNINGS DISTRIBUTION IN THE UNITED STATES, 1969. HEW publication no. (SSA) 75-11914. Washington, D.C.: Government Printing Office, 1974.

        Lists 1969 earnings by age, sex, and race of worker within geographic area of employment. Data for United States, regions, metropolitan, and nonmetropolitan areas.

Appendix A
NEWSLETTERS AND JOURNALS

This appendix includes a brief list of newsletters and a list of journals. The newsletters cited provide data users with information about the state of the art in the collection of vital and health statistics, the use of statistics, and new publications. They principally cover activities of the federal government and are an important service for current information.

Journals cited here have been selected for their frequent publication of statistical articles. Some, such as the AMERICAN JOURNAL OF EPIDEMIOLOGY (see A.5), cover the material almost exclusively while others may have only one or several articles per issue. These journals are fairly common, are indexed in the major health indexes and abstracts, and appear in the computerized bibliographic data bases as well.

NEWSLETTERS

A.1   DATA USER NEWS. U.S. Bureau of the Census, Subscriber Services Section, Washington, D.C. 20233, 1966-- . Monthly.

A.2   NEWS OF THE COOPERATIVE HEALTH STATISTICS SYSTEM. U.S. National Center for Health Statistics, 3700 East-West Highway, Hyattsville, Md. 20852, 1974-- . Bimonthly.

A.3   STATISTICAL NOTES FOR HEALTH PLANNERS. U.S. National Center for Health Statistics, 3700 East-West Highway, Hyattsville, Md. 20852, July 1976-- . Irregular.

A.4   STATISTICAL REPORTER. Superintendent of Documents, Government Printing Office, Washington, D.C. 20402, 1945-- . Monthly.

Newsletters and Journals

JOURNALS

A.5 AMERICAN JOURNAL OF EPIDEMIOLOGY. Johns Hopkins University, School of Hygiene and Public Health, 615 North Wolfe Street, Baltimore, Md. 21205, 1921-- . Monthly.

A.6 AMERICAN JOURNAL OF PUBLIC HEALTH. American Public Health Association, 1015 Eighteenth Street, N.W., Washington, D.C. 20036, 1911-- . Monthly.

A.7 AMERICAN JOURNAL OF TROPICAL MEDICINE AND HYGIENE. American Society of Parasitologists, Box 368, Lawrence, Kans. 66044, 1921-- . Bimonthly.

A.8 ARCHIVES OF ENVIRONMENTAL HEALTH. Heldreff Publications, 4000 Albemarle Street, N.W., Washington, D.C. 20016, 1950-- . Bimonthly.

A.9 BLUE CROSS REPORTS RESEARCH SERIES. Blue Cross Association, 840 North Lake Shore Drive, Chicago, Ill. 60611, 1969-- . 3 or 4 per year.

A.10 DIABETES. American Diabetes Association, 1 West Forty Eighth Street, New York, N.Y. 10020, 1952-- . Monthly.

A.11 DM: DISEASE-A-MONTH. Year Book Medical Publishers, 35 East Wacker Drive, Chicago, Ill. 60601, 1954-- . Monthly.

A.12 HEALTH PLANNING INFORMATION SERIES. Bureau of Health Planning and Resources Development, National Health Planning Information Center, Rockville, Md. 20852, 1976-- . Irregular.

A.13 HEALTH SERVICES RESEARCH. Hospital Research and Educational Trust, 840 North Lake Shore Drive, Chicago, Ill. 60611, 1966-- . Quarterly.

A.14 HOSPITALS, JOURNAL OF THE AMERICAN HOSPITAL ASSOCIATION. American Hospital Association, 840 North Lake Shore Drive, Chicago, Ill. 60611, 1936-- . Semimonthly.

A.15 INQUIRY: A JOURNAL OF MEDICAL CARE ORGANIZATION, PROVISION AND FINANCING. Blue Cross Association, 840 North Lake Shore Drive, Chicago, Ill. 60611, 1963-- . Quarterly.

Newsletters and Journals

A.16 INTERNATIONAL JOURNAL OF EPIDEMIOLOGY. Oxford University Press, 200 Madison Avenue, New York, N.Y. 10016, 1972-- . Quarterly.

A.17 INTERNATIONAL JOURNAL OF HEALTH SERVICES. Baywood Publishing Co., 120 Marine Street, Farmingdale, N.Y. 11735, 1971-- . Quarterly.

A.18 JOURNAL OF CHRONIC DISEASES. Pergamon Press, Headington Hill Hall, Oxford OX3 OBW, Engl., 1955-- . Monthly.

A.19 JOURNAL OF INFECTIOUS DISEASES. University of Chicago Press, 5801 Ellis Avenue, Chicago, Ill. 60637, 1904-- . Monthly.

A.20 JOURNAL OF MEDICAL EDUCATION. Association of American Medical Colleges, One Dupont Circle, N.W., Washington, D.C. 20036, 1926-- . Monthly.

A.21 JOURNAL OF THE NATIONAL CANCER INSTITUTE. Superintendent of Documents, Government Printing Office, Washington, D.C. 20402, 1940-- . Monthly.

A.22 JOURNAL OF OCCUPATIONAL MEDICINE. American Occupational Medical Association, North Wacker Drive, Chicago, Ill. 60606, 1959-- . Monthly.

A.23 JOURNAL OF STUDIES ON ALCOHOL. Journal of Studies on Alcohol, Center of Alcohol Studies, Rutgers University, The State University of New Jersey, New Brunswick, N.J. 08903, 1940-- . Monthly.

A.24 MEDICAL CARE. (American Public Health Association) J.B. Lippincott Co., East Washington Square, Philadelphia, Pa. 19105, 1967-- . Monthly.

A.25 MEDICAL ECONOMICS. Medical Economics Co., Oradell, N.J. 07649, 1923-- . Biweekly.

A.26 MILBANK MEMORIAL FUND QUARTERLY, HEALTH & SOCIETY. 156 Fifth Avenue, Room 502, New York, N.Y. 10010, 1923-- .

A.27 PAS REPORTER. Commission on Professional and Hospital Activities, 1968 Green Road, Ann Arbor, Mich. 48105, Irregular.

Newsletters and Journals

A.28 PREVENTIVE MEDICINE. Academic Press, 111 Fifth Avenue, New York, N.Y. 10003, 1972-- . Quarterly.

A.29 PUBLIC HEALTH REPORTS. Superintendent of Documents, Government Printing Office, Washington, D.C. 20402, 1974-- . Monthly.

A.30 SOCIAL SECURITY BULLETIN. Superintendent of Documents, Government Printing Office, Washington, D.C. 20402, 1938-- . Monthly.

A.31 STATISTICAL BULLETIN. Metropolitan Life Insurance Co., 1 Madison Avenue, New York, N.Y., 1920-- . Monthly.

A.32 TOPICS IN HEALTH CARE FINANCING. Aspen Systems Corp., 11600 Nebel Street, Rockville, Md. 20852, 1974-- . Quarterly.

Appendix B
GOVERNMENT AGENCIES

Government agencies are probably the most important source for health statistics users. As is evident in the bibliography, government agencies are responsible for the collection and dissemination of vital statistics as well as for many other types of health statistics. This section is divided into lists of state, federal, and international agencies. Refer to the NATIONAL DIRECTORY OF STATE AGENCIES (see no. 1.26), the UNITED STATES GOVERNMENT MANUAL (see no. 1.23), THE NATIONAL HEALTH DIRECTORY (see no. 1.19a), and the MEDICAL AND HEALTH INFORMATION DIRECTORY (see no. 1.19) for more complete listings.

STATE AGENCIES

Publications of state agencies have not been included in this bibliography, but sources of their publications have. (See no. 1.34 and no. 1.37.) Presented here is the address and telephone number of the major health department in each state.

B.1   ALABAMA: Division of Public Health, State Office Building, 501 Dexter Avenue, Montgomery, Ala. 36130. (205) 832-3120

B.2   ALASKA: Division of Public Health, Department of Health and Social Services, 503 Alaska Office Building, 350 Main Street, Pouch H-06, Juneau, Alaska 99811. (907) 465-3090

B.3   AMERICAN SAMOA: Department of Medical Services, Office of the Governor, LBJ Tropical Medical Center, Pago Pago, Samoa 96799 633-4116

B.4   ARIZONA: Department of Health Services, 1740 West Adams Street, Phoenix, Ariz. 85007. (602) 271-3113

Government Agencies

B.5 ARKANSAS: Department of Health, 4815 West Markham Street, Little Rock, Ark. 72201. (501) 661-2111

B.6 CALIFORNIA: Department of Health, State Office Building 8, 714 P Street, Sacramento, Calif. 95814. (916) 445-1248

B.7 COLORADO: Department of Health, 4210 East Eleventh Avenue, Denver, Colo. 80220. (303) 388-6111, Ext. 315

B.8 CONNECTICUT: Department of Health, 79 Elm Street, Hartford, Conn. 06115. (203) 566-2279

B.9 DELAWARE: Divison of Public Health, Department of Health and Social Services, Jesse S. Cooper Memorial Building, Dover, Del. 19901. (302) 678-4701

B.10 DISTRICT OF COLUMBIA: Community Health and Hospitals Administration, Department of Human Resources, 1875 Connecticut Avenue, N.W., Washington, D.C. 20009. (202) 629-3366

B.11 FLORIDA: Health Program Office, Department of Health and Rehabilitative Services, 1323 Winewood Boulevard, Tallahassee, Fla. 32301. (904) 488-4115

B.12 GEORGIA: Division of Physical Health, Department of Human Resources, 522 Health Building, 47 Trinity Avenue, S.W., Atlanta, Ga. 30334. (404) 656-4655

B.13 GUAM: Department of Public Health and Social Services, P.O. Box 2816, Agana, Guam 96910. 734-9917

B.14 HAWAII: Department of Health, Kinau Hale, 1250 Punchbowl Street, P.O. Box 3378 (96801), Honolulu, Hawaii 96813. (808) 548-6505

B.15 IDAHO: Division of Health, Department of Health and Welfare, State Office Building, 700 West State Street, Boise, Idaho 83720. (208) 384-3401

B.16 ILLINOIS: Department of Public Health, 525 West Jefferson Street, Springfield, Ill. 62706. (217) 782-4977

B.17 INDIANA: Board of Health, 425 Health Building, 1330 West Michigan Street, Indianapolis, Ind. 46206. (317) 633-5490

Government Agencies

B.18　IOWA: Department of Health, Robert Lucas State Office Building, East Twelfth and Walnut Streets, Des Moines, Iowa 50319. (515) 281-5605

B.19　KANSAS: Department of Health and Environment, Building 740, Forbes Air Force Base, Topeka, Kans. 66620. (913) 296-3745

B.20　KENTUCKY: Bureau for Health Services, Department for Human Resources, Health Building, 275 East Main Street, Frankfurt, Ky. 40601. (502) 564-3970

B.21　LOUISIANA: Health and Human Resources Administration, State Office Building, 150 Riverside Mall, Baton Rouge, La. 70801. (504) 389-5796

B.22　MAINE: Bureau of Health, Department of Human Services, State House, Augusta, Maine 04333. (207) 289-3201

B.23　MARYLAND: Department of Health and Mental Hygiene, Herbert R. O'Conor State Office Building, 201 West Preston Street, Baltimore, Md. 21201. (301) 383-6195

B.24　MASSACHUSETTS: Department of Public Health, 600 Washington Street, Boston, Mass. 02111. (617) 727-2700

B.25　MICHIGAN: Department of Public Health, 3500 North Logan Street, Lansing, Mich. 48909. (517) 373-1320

B.26　MINNESOTA: Department of Health, State Board of Health Building, 717 Delaware Street, S.E., Minneapolis, Minn. 55440. (612) 296-5460

B.27　MISSISSIPPI: Mississippi State Board of Health, 2423 North State Street, P.O. Box 1700, Jackson, Miss. 39205. (601) 354-6646

B.28　MISSOURI: Division of Health, Department of Social Services, Broadway State Office Building, High Street and Broadway, P.O. Box 570, Jefferson City, Mo. 65101. (314) 751-4330

B.29　MONTANA: Department of Health and Environmental Sciences, 200 W.F. Cogswell Building, Lockey Street, Helena, Mont. 59601. (406) 449-2544

B.30　NEBRASKA: Department of Health, Lincoln Building, 2d Floor, 1003 O Street, Lincoln, Nebr. 68508. (402) 471-2133

Government Agencies

B.31 NEVADA: Health Division, Department of Human Resources, Kinkead Building, 505 East King Street, Capitol Complex, Carson City, Nev. 89710. (702) 885-4740

B.32 NEW HAMPSHIRE: Division of Public Health, Department of Health and Welfare, 61 South Spring Street, Concord, N.H. 03301. (603) 271-2526

B.33 NEW JERSEY: Department of Health, John Fitch Plaza, P.O. Box 1540, Trenton, N.J. 08625. (609) 292-7837

B.34 NEW MEXICO: State Health Agency, Department of Health and Social Services, Crown State Office Building, 725 St. Michaels Drive, P.O. Box 2348, Sante Fe, N. Mex. 87503. (505) 827-3201

B.35 NEW YORK: Department of Health, Tower Building, Empire State Plaza, Albany, N.Y. 12237. (518) 474-2011

B.36 NORTH CAROLINA: Division of Health Services, Department of Human Resources, 225 North McDowell Street, P.O. Box 2091, Raleigh, N.C. 27602. (919) 829-3446

B.37 NORTH DAKOTA: Department of Health, State Capitol, Bismarck, N. Dak. 58505. (701) 224-2371

B.38 OHIO: Department of Health, 450 East Town Street, Columbus, Ohio 43215. (614) 466-2253

B.39 OKLAHOMA: Department of Health, North East Tenth and Stonewall Streets, P.O. Box 53551, Oklahoma City, Okla. 73105. (405) 271-4200

B.40 OREGON: Health Division, Department of Human Resources, 930 State Office Building, 1400 South West Fifth Avenue, P.O. Box 231, Portland, Oreg. 97201. (503) 229-5032

B.41 PENNSYLVANIA: Department of Health, 802 Health and Welfare Building, P.O. Box 90, Harrisburg, Pa. 17120. (717) 787-6436

B.42 PUERTO RICO: Department of Health, 1306 Ponce de Leon Avenue, P.O. Box 9342, Santurce, P.R. 00908. (809) 724-6387 and 723-6323

B.43 RHODE ISLAND: Department of Health, 401 State Health Department Building, 75 Davis Street, Providence, R.I. 02908. (401) 277-2231

Government Agencies

B.44 SOUTH CAROLINA: Department of Health and Environmental Control, R.J. Aycock Building, 2600 Bull Street, Columbia, S.C. 29201. (803) 758-5443

B.45 SOUTH DAKOTA: Department of Health, Joe Foss Building, Pierre, S. Dak. 57501. (605) 224-3361

B.46 TENNESSEE: Department of Public Health, Cordell Hull Building, 436 Sixth Avenue, N., Nashville, Tenn. 37219. (615) 741-3111.

B.47 TEXAS: Department of Health Resources, 1100 West Forty Ninth Street, Austin, Tex. 78756. (512) 454-3781

B.48 UTAH: Division of Health, Department of Social Services, 44 Medical Drive, Salt Lake City, Utah 84113. (801) 533-6111

B.49 VERMONT: Department of Health, 60 Main Street, Burlington, Vt. 05401. (802) 862-5701

B.50 VIRGINIA: Department of Health, James Madison Building, 109 Governor Street, Richmond, Va. 23219. (804) 786-3561

B.51 VIRGIN ISLANDS: Department of Health, Government House, Charlotte Amalie, St. Thomas, V.I. 00801. (809) 774-0117

B.52 WASHINGTON: Health Services Division, Department of Social and Health Sciences, Mail Stop 444, Olympia, Wash. 98504. (206) 753-5871

B.53 WEST VIRGINIA: Department of Health, 535 State Office Building, 1800 Washington Street, E., Charleston, W. Va. 25305. (304) 348-2971

B.54 WISCONSIN: Division of Health, Department of Health and Social Services, 434 Wilson Street State Office Building, 1 West Wilson Street, P.O. Box 309, Madison, Wis. 53701. (608) 266-1511

B.55 WYOMING: Department of Health and Social Services, Hataway Building, 2300 Capitol Avenue, Cheyenne, Wyo. 82002. (307) 777-7657

Government Agencies

FEDERAL AGENCIES

The agencies presented here include information clearinghouses as well as agencies which collect and publish statistics. Check the index for specific publications. All agencies listed will provide publications or information upon request. Incidentally, it should be noted that federal agencies change addresses, telephone numbers, and even names quite frequently. The information given here is current at this time.

Several important sources for health statistics should be pointed out since they provide quite extensive reference services. These are: (1) the U.S. National Center for Health Statistics (see B.74), (2) the U.S. National Health Planning Information Center (see B.81), (3) the U.S. Bureau of the Census (see B.60), and (4) NTIS Statistical Data Reference Service (see B.91). The last provides services for a substantial fee only, while the others provide free services.

B.56 Bureau of Community Health Service, Office for Maternal and Child Health Services, 5600 Fishers Lane, Rockville, Md. 20857. (301) 443-4273

B.57 Bureau of Health Manpower, Health Resources Administration, Prince George's Center, 3700 East-West Highway, Hyattsville, Md. 20782. (301) 436-6448

B.58 Bureau of Health Planning Methods and Technology, Health Resources Administration, 3700 East-West Highway, Hyattsville, Md. 20782. (301) 436-6110

B.59 Bureau of Labor Statistics, Consumer Price Index, 441 G Street, N.W., Washington, D.C. 20212. (202) 523-1222

B.60 Bureau of the Census, Population Division, Department of Commerce, Washington, D.C. 20233. (301) 763-5002

B.61 Cancer Information Clearinghouse, 7910 Woodmont Avenue, Bethesda, Md. 20014. (301) 496-4070

B.62 Center for Disease Control, Atlanta, Ga. 30333. (404) 633-3311

B.63 Clearinghouse on Health Indexes, National Center for Health Statistics, Prince George's Center Building, 3700 East-West Highway, Hyattsville, Md. 20782. (301) 436-7035

B.64 Clearinghouse on the Handicapped, Office of Handicapped Individuals, Room 388-D, South Portal Building, Washington, D.C. 20201. (202) 245-1961

Government Agencies

B.65 Consumer Product Safety Commission, National Injury Information Clearinghouse, Westwood Building, 5401 Westbard Avenue, Bethesda, Md. 20207. (301) 492-6424

B.66 Diabetes Information Clearinghouse, National Institute for Arthritis, Metabolism and Digestive Diseases, 9000 Rockville Pike, Bethesda, Md. 20014. (301) 496-7418

B.67 Division of Nursing, Bureau of Health Manpower, Prince George's Center, 3700 East-West Highway, Hyattsville, Md. 20782. (301) 436-6624

B.68 End-Stage Renal Disease Program, Health Care Financing Administration, 5600 Fishers Lane, Rockville, Md. 20857. (301) 443-3617

B.69 Health Care Financing Administration, Office of Policy Planning and Research, 330 C Street, S.W., Washington, D.C. 20201. (202) 245-0340 (Medicaid); (202) 472-3705 (Medicare)

B.70 Indian Health Service, 5600 Fishers Lane, Room 6A-30, Rockville, Md. 20857. (301) 443-1180

B.71 Maternal and Child Health Service, Health Services Administration, 5600 Fishers Lane, Rockville, Md. 20857. (301) 443-4273

B.72 National Cancer Institute, Office of Cancer Communications, Building 31, Room 10 A-18, 9000 Rockville Pike, Bethesda Md., 20014. (301) 496-6641

B.73 National Center for Education Statistics, 400 Maryland Avenue, S.W., Washington, D.C. 20202. (202) 245-8795

B.74 National Center for Health Statistics, Scientific and Technical Information Branch, Prince George's Center, 3700 East-West Highway, Hyattsville, Md. 20782. (301) 436-8500

B.75 National Clearinghouse for Alcohol Information, P.O. Box 1126, Rockville, Md. 20850. (301) 948-4450

B.76 National Clearinghouse for Mental Health Information, National Institute of Mental Health, 5600 Fishers Lane, Rockville, Md. 20857. (301) 443-4517

Government Agencies

B.77   National Clearinghouse for Smoking and Health, Center for Disease Control, Atlanta, Ga. 30333. (404) 633-3311

B.78   National Clearinghouse on Aging, Administration on Aging, Room 4552, HEW North Building, 330 Independence Avenue, S.W., Washington, D.C. 20201. (202) 245-0768

B.79   National Clearinghouse on Drug Abuse, Alcohol, Drug Abuse, and Mental Health Information, 5600 Fishers Lane, Rockville, Md. 20857. (301) 443-6500

B.80   National Eye Institute, Building 31, Room 6 A-25, 9000 Rockville Pike, Bethesda, Md. 20014. (301) 496-5248

B.81   National Health Planning Information Center, Prince George's Center, 3700 East-West Highway, Hyattsville, Md. 20782. (301) 436-6733

B.82   National Heart and Lung Institute, Federal Building, Room 200, 7550 Wisconsin Avenue, Bethesda, Md. 20014. (301) 496-5826

B.83   National Institute of Arthritis, Metabolism, and Digestive Diseases, Office of Scientific and Technical Reports, Building 31, Room 9A-04, 9000 Rockville Pike, Bethesda, Md. 20014. (301) 496-3583

B.84   National Institute of Child Health and Human Development, 9000 Rockville Pike, Bethesda, Md. 20014. (301) 496-5133

B.85   National Institute of Dental Research, Dental Research Data Office, Westwood Building, 5333 Westbard Avenue, Bethesda, Md. 20016. (301) 496-7220

B.86   National Institute of Mental Health, 5600 Fishers Lane, Rockville, Md. 20857. (301) 443-3683

B.87   National Institute of Neurological and Communicative Disorders and Stroke, Building 31, Room 8A-06, 9000 Rockville Pike, Rockville, Md. 20014. (301) 496-4106

B.88   National Institute on Drug Abuse, Division of Scientific and Program Information, Room 105, 11400 Rockville Pike, Rockville, Md. 20852. (301) 443-6637

Government Agencies

B.89   National Institutes of Health Publications, Building 31, Room 2B03, 9000 Rockville Pike, Bethesda, Md. 20014. (301) 496-4143

B.90   National Technical Information Service, U.S. Department of Commerce, Springfield, Va. 22161. (202) 724-3382 (publication information) or (703) 557-4642 (NTIS searches)

B.91   NTIS Statistical Data Reference Service (fee for service), c/o DUALabs, Suite 900, 1601 North Kent Street, Arlington, Va. 22209. (703) 525-1480, ext. 95

B.92   Occupational Safety and Health Statistics, Bureau of Labor Statistics, U.S. Department of Labor, Washington, D.C. 20210. (202) 523-9275

B.93   President's Committee on Mental Retardation, Regional Office Building, Seventh and D Streets, S.W., Washington, D.C. 20201. (202) 245-7634

B.94   Public Health Service Publications, Room 745G, 200 Independence Avenue, S.W., Washington, D.C. 20201. (202) 245-6867

B.95   Social Security Administration, 6401 Security Boulevard, 100 Altmeyer Building, Baltimore, Md. 21235. (301) 594-2883

B.96   Social Security Administration, Division of Disability Studies, Room 3C2, Meadows East, Baltimore, Md. 21235. (301) 594-0304

B.97   Social Security Administration, Office of Research and Statistics, 1875 Connecticut Avenue, N.W., Washington, D.C. 20009. (202) 673-5614

B.98   Superintendent of Documents, Government Printing Office, Washington, D.C. 20402. (202) 783-3238 (publication information)

INTERNATIONAL AGENCIES

B.99   International Agency for Research on Cancer (IARC), 150 Cours Albert-Thomas, F-69009 Lyon, France

B.100   Pan American Health Organization (PAHO), Twenty Third Street, N.W., Washington, D.C. 20037. (202) 223-4700

B.101   United Nations (UN), UN Publications (LX 2300), New York, N.Y. 10017

Government Agencies

B.102 World Health Organization (WHO), Distribution and Sales Service, CH-1211 Geneva 27, Switz. (For subscriptions only; the U.S. distributor for single and bulk copies of WHO publications is: Q Corporation, P.O. Box 433, Murray Hill Station, New York, N.Y. 10016.

Appendix C
ASSOCIATIONS

Associations and research organizations are a rich source of health statistics. This section includes those which publish information and those which have unpublished information available. The name, address, and telephone number for each is given.

Refer to the index for cited publications by these associations. The ENCYCLOPEDIA OF ASSOCIATIONS (see no. 1.17) is a comprehensive source for further information about these associations.

C.1 American Burn Association
New York Hospital-Cornell
   Medical Center
Room F0758
525 East Sixty-eighth Street
New York, New York 10021
(212) 744-4447

C.2 American Cancer Society
777 Third Avenue
New York, N.Y. 10017
(212) 371-2900, ext. 401

C.3 American College of Surgeons
55 East Erie Street
Chicago, Ill. 60611
(312) 664-4050

C.4 American Dental Association
211 East Chicago Avenue
Chicago, Ill. 60611
(312) 944-6730

C.5 American Diabetes Association
600 Fifth Avenue
New York, N.Y. 10020
(212) 541-4310

C.6 American Heart Association
7320 Greenville Avenue
Dallas, Tex. 75231
(214) 750-5300

C.7 American Hospital Association
840 North Lake Shore Drive
Chicago, Ill. 60611
(312) 645-9400

C.8 American Nurses' Association
2420 Pershing Road
Kansas City, Mo. 64108
(816) 474-5720

C.9 Arthritis Foundation
3400 Peachtree Road, N.E.
Suite 1101,
Atlanta, Ga. 30326
(404) 266-0795

C.10 Association of American Medical
   Colleges
One Dupont Circle, N.W.
Washington, D.C. 20036
(202) 466-5100

Associations

C.11 Blue Cross Association,
840 North Lake Shore Dirve,
Chicago, Ill. 60611.
(312) 440-6000

C.12 Commission on Professional and
Hospital Activities
1968 Green Road
Ann Arbor, Mich. 48105
(313) 769-6511

C.13 Committee to Combat Huntington's Disease
250 West Fifty-seventh Street,
Suite 2016
New York, N.Y. 10019
(212) 757-9443

C.14 Epilepsy Foundation of America
1828 L Street, N.W., Suite 406
Washington, D.C. 20036
(202) 293-2930

C.15 Health Insurance Institute
1850 K Street, N.W.
Washington, D.C. 20006
(202) 393-3041

C.16 Infectious Diseases Society of America
C/O Dr. Theodore C. Eickhoff
Box B-168
University of Colorado Medical Center
Denver, Colo. 80262
(303) 394-7233

C.17 Muscular Dystrophy Association
810 Seventh Avenue
New York, N.Y. 10019
(212) 586-0808

C.18 Myasthenia Gravis Foundation
15 East Twenty-sixth Street
New York, New York 10010
(212) 889-8157

C.19 National ALS Foundation
185 Madison Avenue
New York, N.Y. 10016
(212) 679-4016

C.20 National Association of the Deaf
814 Thayer Avenue
Silver Spring, Md. 20910
(301) 587-1788

C.21 National Center for Child Abuse and Neglect
400 Sixth Street, S.W.
Washington, D.C. 20201
(202) 755-8208

C.22 National Dialysis Registry
Artificial Kidney-Chronic Uremia Program of the National Institute of Arthritis and Metabolic Diseases
National Institutes of Health
9000 Rockville Pike
Bethesda, Md. 20014
(301) 496-7459

C.23 National Foundation, March of Dimes
1275 Mamaronick Avenue
White Plains, New York 10605
(914) 428-7100

C.24 National League for Nursing
Ten Columbus Circle
New York, N.Y. 10019
(212) 582-1022

C.25 National Multiple Sclerosis Society
205 East Forty Second Street
New York, N.Y. 10017
(212) 986-3240

C.26 National Safety Council
444 North Michigan Avenue
Chicago, Ill. 60611
(312) 527-4800

Associations

C.27 National Sudden Infant Death Syndrome Foundation
310 South Michigan Avenue
Chicago, Ill. 60604
(312) 663-0650

C.28 Population Reference Bureau
1337 Connecticut Avenue, N.W.
Washington, D.C. 20036
(202) 785-4664

C.29 Sickle Cell Disease Foundation of Greater New York
209 West 125th Street
Room 108
New York, N.Y. 10027
(212) 850-1920

C.30 United Cerebral Palsy Associations
66 East Thirty-fourth Street
New York, N.Y. 10016
(212) 481-6300

Appendix D
REGIONAL DEPOSITORY LIBRARIES

Since many sources of health data are government publications, a list of regional depository libraries has been provided here.

Health sciences libraries may not have extensive document collections even in the medical and health-related subjects because of the elusive nature of these publications. Regional depositories have comprehensive collections and must by law make them available to the public.

The DIRECTORY OF GOVERNMENT DOCUMENT COLLECTIONS AND LIBRARIANS (see no. 1.16) should be consulted for more detailed information about document collections and their availability.

D.1 ALABAMA
Auburn University of Montgomery Library
Montgomery, Ala. 36117
(205) 279-9110, ext. 251

D.2 University of Alabama Library
Box S
University, Ala. 35486
(205) 348-6045

D.3 ARIZONA
Arizona Department of Library, Archives and Public Records
3rd Floor, Capitol
Phoenix, Ariz. 85007
(602) 271-3701

D.4 University of Arizona Library
Government Documents Department
Tucson, Ariz. 85721
(602) 884-4871

D.5 CALIFORNIA
California State Library
Government Publications Section
P.O. Box 2037
Sacramento, Calif. 95809
(916) 322-4572

D.6 COLORADO
University of Colorado at Boulder Norlin Library
Government Documents Division
Boulder, Colo. 80309
(303) 492-8834

Regional Depository Libraries

D.7 CONNECTICUT
Connecticut State Library
231 Capitol Avenue
Hartford, Conn. 06115
(203) 544-4971

D.8 FLORIDA
University of Florida
Library West
Documents Department
Gainesville, Fla. 32611
(904) 392-0367

D.9 GEORGIA
University of Georgia
University Libraries
Government Reference
Athens, Ga. 30602
(404) 542-8949

D.10 HAWAII
University of Hawaii, Manoa
Library, Government Documents
Collection
2425 Campus Road
Honolulu, Hawaii 96822
(808) 948-8230

D.11 IDAHO
University of Idaho Library
Social Science Library
Moscow, Idaho 83843
(208) 885-6344

D.12 ILLINOIS
Illinois State Library
Documents Branch
Centennial Building
Springfield, Ill. 62756
(217) 782-5185

D.13 INDIANA
Indiana State Library
140 North Senate Avenue
Indianapolis, Ind. 46204
(317) 633-6425

D.14 IOWA
University of Iowa
Libraries
Government Publications Department
Iowa City, Iowa 52242
(319) 353-3318

D.15 KANSAS
University of Kansas
Watson Library
Lawrence, Kans. 66044
(913) 864-4662

D.16 KENTUCKY
University of Kentucky
Margaret I. King Library
Government Publications Department
Lexington, Ky. 40506
(606) 257-2639

D.17 LOUISIANA
Louisiana State University
Library
Baton Rouge, La. 70803
(504) 388-2570

D.18 MAINE
University of Maine at Orono
Raymond H. Fogler Library
Orono, Maine 04473
(207) 581-7178

D.19 MARYLAND
University of Maryland
McKeldin Library
College Park, Md. 20742
(301) 454-3034

D.20 MASSACHUSETTS
Boston Public Library
Government Documents Department
Copley Square
Boston, Mass. 02117
(617) 535-5400, ext. 295

Regional Depository Libraries

D.21 MICHIGAN
Detroit Public Library
5201 Woodward Avenue
Detroit, Mich. 48202
(313) 321-1409

D.22 Michigan State Library
Documents Library
525 West Ottawa Street
Lansing, Mich. 48909
(517) 373-0640

D.23 MINNESOTA
University of Minnesota
O. Meredith Wilson Library
Government Publications Division
409 Wilson Library
Minneapolis, Minn. 55455
(612) 373-7813

D.24 MISSISSIPPI
University of Mississippi
Library
University, Miss. 38677
(601) 232-7091

D.25 MONTANA
University of Montana
Library
Missoula, Mont. 59812
(406) 243-6700

D.26 NEBRASKA
Nebraska Library Commission
Nebraska Publications Clearinghouse
1420 P Street
Lincoln, Nebr. 68508
(402) 471-2045

D.27 NEVADA
University of Nevada, Reno
Library,
Government Publications Department
Reno, Nev. 89557
(702) 784-6579

D.28 NEW JERSEY
Newark Public Library
Lending and Reference Department
5 Washington Street
Newark, N.J. 07101
(201) 733-7740

D.29 NEW MEXICO
New Mexico State Library
300 Don Gasper
Santa Fe, N. Mex. 87501
(505) 827-2033

D.30 University of New Mexico
Zimmerman Library
Government Publications
Section
Albuquerque, N. Mex. 97131
(505) 277-5441

D.31 NEW YORK
New York State Library
Education Building
Albany, N.Y. 12234
(518) 474-5563

D.32 NORTH CAROLINA
University of North Carolina
at Chapel Hill
Louis Round Wilson Library
024-A
BAISS Division
Chapel Hill, N.C. 27514
(919) 933-1551

D.33 NORTH DAKOTA
North Dakota State University
Library, Documents Office
Fargo, N. Dak. 58102
(701) 237-8876

D.34 OHIO
State Library of Ohio
65 South Front Street
Columbus, Ohio 43215
(614) 466-2694

Regional Depository Libraries

D.35 OKLAHOMA
Oklahoma Department of
Libraries
200 Northeast Eighteenth Street
Oklahoma City, Okla. 73105
(405) 521-2502

D.36 OREGON
Portland State University
Library
P.O. Box 1151
Portland, Oreg. 97207
(503) 229-3673

D.37 PENNSYLVANIA
State Library of Pennsylvania
Government Publications
Section
P.O. Box 1601
Harrisburg, Pa. 17126
(717) 787-3752

D.38 TEXAS
Texas State Library
P.O. Box 12927
Capitol Station
Austin, Tex. 78711
(512) 475-2996

D.39 Texas Tech University Library
Documents Department
P.O. Box 4079
Lubbock, Tex. 79409
(806) 742-2268

D.40 UTAH
Utah State University
Merrill Library
Government Documents Department
Logan, Utah 84322
(801) 752-7554

D.41 VIRGINIA
University of Virginia
Alderman Library
Charlottesville, Va. 22901
(804) 924-3516

D.42 WASHINGTON
Washington State Library
Olympia, Wash. 98504
(206) 753-4394

D.43 WEST VIRGINIA
West Virginia University
Library
Morgantown, W. Va. 26506
(305) 293-5395

D.44 WISCONSIN
Milwaukee Public Library
Central Library
814 West Wisconsin Avenue
Milwaukee, Wis. 53233
(414) 278-3000

D.45 WYOMING
Wyoming State Library
Documents Section
Information Services Division
Supreme Court and Library
Building
Cheyenne, Wyo. 82002
(307) 777-7281, ext. 21

Appendix E
SUPPLIERS OF BIBLIOGRAPHIC DATA FILES

The organizations listed below may be contacted directly for information on specific prices and conditions of access to their data bases.

E.1 Bibliographic Retrieval Services (BRS)
Corporations Park, Building 702
Scotia, N.Y. 12302
(518) 374-5011

E.2 Lockheed Information Systems
Orgn. 5208, Building 201
3251 Hanover Street
Palo Alto, Calif. 94304
(800) 227-1960

E.3 National Library of Medicine (NLM)
8600 Rockville Pike
Bethesda, Md. 20014
(301) 496-6193

E.4 SDC Search Service
2500 Colorado Avenue
Santa Monica, Calif. 90406
(203) 829-7511

GLOSSARY

Age-adjusted rate
: Used to compare two population groups in which the age distribution differs. To compare the two populations, the age-specific rates for each population are applied to a selected standard population.

Age-specific birth rate
: The number of live births to women in a selected age group per 1,000 women in that same age group.

Age-specific death rate
: The number of deaths reported in a selected age group per 1,000 population in that same age group.

Average daily census
: Average number of inpatients present each day during a given period of time.

Cause-specific death rate
: The number of deaths from a specific cause in a calendar year per 1,000 population.

Chronic disease
: Diseases which have one or more of the following characteristics: (1) are permanent, (2) leave a disability, (3) are caused by nonreversible pathological alteration, (4) require special training of the patient for rehabilitation, (5) may be expected to require a long period of supervision, observation or care.

Cohort study
: An inquiry in which a group (the cohort) is chosen for the presence of a specific characteristic at a specified time and followed over a period of time for the appearance of related characteristics; e.g., a group of diabetics followed to check the appearance of heart or renal disease.

Communicable disease
: An illness resulting from the spread or transmission of an infectious agent.

Glossary

Crude birth rate	The number of live births in a calendar year per 1,000 population.
Crude death rate	The number of deaths reported in a calendar year per 1,000 population.
Demography	Statistical study of human populations with emphasis on size, density, distribution, and composition.
Fertility rate	The number of live births per 1,000 women aged 15-44.
Health status indicator	A statistic that generally reflects the health of a specific population when compared to the total population.
Incidence rate	The number of new cases of disease which occur during a particular time period in a particular population.
Infant mortality rate	The number of deaths of infants under one year of age during a calendar year per 1,000 live births.
Length of stay	This is determined by subtracting the date of admission from the date of discharge.
Life table	A mathematical model that portrays mortality conditions among a population and provides a basis for measuring longevity. With a life table one can determine: (a) the probability of dying within one year of a person's life at each age, (b) the average number of years a newborn can expect to live, (c) the average number of years remaining to a person at any age, (d) the probability of surviving from one age to another, (e) the probability of surviving for any given number of years for a person at any age.
Live birth	The complete expulsion or extrication from its mother of a product of conception, irrespective of the duration of pregnancy, which after such separation, breathes or shows other evidence of life whether or not the umbilical cord has been cut.
Maternal mortality rate	The number of maternal deaths attributed to puerperal causes per 1,000 live births.
Morbidity	The extent of illness, injury or disability in a defined population. This is usually expressed in incidence or prevalence rates.
Mortality	Death, usually expressed in rates.

Glossary

Natality	Birth, usually expressed in rates.
Neonatal mortality rate	Deaths under 28 days of age per 1,000 population.
Patient discharge days	The total number of days of care received in an institution by the individuals who were discharged during a given time period.
Perinatal mortality rate	The number of still births plus neonatal deaths per 1,000 total births.
Population at risk	That segment of the population that is vulnerable to a specific health problem.
Postneonatal mortality rate	The number of deaths which occur between the ages of 28 days and one year of age per 1,000 total live births.
Prevalence rate	The number of cases of a given illness at a particular time per 100,000 population.
Socioeconomic status	An individual's position in a given society as determined by factors such as wealth, occupation, and social class.
Standard Metropolitan Statistical Area (SMSA)	A county or group of contiguous counties which contain at least one city of 50,000 population or more.
Stillbirth	This is a synonym for the fetal death that occurs in latter periods of pregnancy.
Vital statistics	Statistics pertaining to births, deaths, fetal deaths, marriage, and divorce.

AUTHOR INDEX

This index includes all authors, editors, compilers, translators, and contributors cited in the text. References are to entry numbers and alphabetization is letter by letter.

A

Ackroyd, Ted J. 1.43
Akey, Denise 1.17
Alan Guttmacher Institute 5.1
Alderson, Michael 1.1
Allen, Gene P. 1.26
Altenfelder, Marion 4.9-.10
American Council of Life Insurance 6.1
American Dental Association 4.11, 4.41, 6.2-.3
American Hospital Association 4.1-.2, 5.2
American Library Association. Government Documents Round Table 1.16
American Medical Association 1.94, 4.12, 4.42, 5.3, 6.4-.5
American Nurses' Association 4.14
American Public Health Association 1.95
Anderson, Odin W. 5.6
Anderson, Ronald 5.4
Andrews, Theodora 1.44
Andriot, John L. 1.32
Arnoff, Franklyn N. 4.15
Association of American Medical Colleges 4.43
Axelrod, S.J. 1.96
Axtell, Lillian M. 3.24

B

Barker, D.J.P. 1.2
Bernero, Jacqueline 1.25
Berry, Ralph E. 6.6
Bourke, Geoffrey J. 1.3
Bridbord, Kenneth 3.14
Buckland, William R. 1.28
Bunker, J.P. 3.6
Burton, Lloyd Edward 1.4

C

Commission on Physicians for the Future 4.44
Commission on Professional and Hospital Activities 5.5
Comprehensive Health Planning Agency of Southeastern Wisconsin 1.27
Consumer Product Safety Commission 3.7
Cooper, Barbara S. 6.7-.9
Culyer, A.J. 1.45

D

Doll, Richard 3.15
Donabedian, A. 1.96
Duncan, Robert C. 1.5
Dyckman, Zachary Y. 6.21

Author Index

E

Efron, Vera 3.10

F

Farlee, Coralie 4.45
Fisher, Charles R. 6.10
Frank, Nathalie D. 1.46
Friedman, Gary D. 1.6

G

Gentry, D.W. 1.96
Gibson, Robert M. 6.10
Goodman, Louis J. 4.16
Grant, Murray 1.7
Grove, Robert D. 2.1, 2.2
Guriolo, C. 3.10

H

Hambleton, Robert 4.22
Health Insurance Institute 6.11
Heinze, Evelyn B. 3.16
Hetzel, Alice M. 2.1
Hill, Sir Austin Bradford 1.8
Hoffstein, Paul A. 6.25
Hu, Teh-wei 6.12
Hudson, Helen H. 4.17

I

Institute of Medicine 6.13
International Agency for Research on Cancer 1.18

J

Jensen, Marilyn Anne 1.47
Jolly, H.P. 4.18

K

Kahn, H.A. 3.55
Keller, Mark 3.10
Kendall, Maurice G. 1.28
Kilpatrick, S. James 1.9
Knopf, Lucille 4.19
Koleda, Michael 6.14
Kruzas, Anthony T. 1.19
Kumbor, A.H. 4.15

L

Lancaster, H.O. 1.10
Larson, Thomas A. 4.45
Levenson, Louis 1.100
Lilienfeld, Abraham M. 1.11
Lindner, Forrest E. 2.2
Livanga, S.K. 1.12
Lowe, C.R. 1.12
Lowell, Anthony N. 3.51
Lufburrow, Nancy C. 1.48

M

McCall, Nelda 6.19
Macdonald, Eleanor J. 3.16
McGilvray, James 1.3
Marquis, Kent 6.15
Moorhead, H.B. 3.55
Mueller, Marjorie Smith 6.15

N

National Health Education Committee 1.98, 3.57
National League for Nursing 4.46
National Safety Council 3.8
Newman, John F. 5.6

O

Oreglia, Anthony 1.29
Ott, Mary D. 4.50

P

Pharmaceutical Manufacturers Association 6.16
Phillips, David A. 1.13
Piore, Nora 5.7

R

Rice, Dorothy P. 6.8, 6.17
Roddy, Pamela C. 4.22
Rowland, Howard S. 1.99a
Rufener, Brent L. 6.18

S

Sartwell, Phillip E. 1.14
Sax, Ellen 1.49

Author Index

Schein, Jerome D. 3.56
Scitovsky, Anne A. 5.8, 6.19
Silberg, Nancy 1.51
Silverberg, Edwin 3.17
Singer, Richard B. 1.100
Smith, Hugh Hollingsworth 1.4
Snyder, Nelda M. 5.8
Strahon, Genevieve W. 4.6

U

United Nations. Statistical Office 1.104-5
U.S. Bureau of Community Health Services 2.3, 3.57a
U.S. Bureau of Health Manpower 1.52, 4.20-.25, 4.26, 4.47-.48
U.S. Bureau of Health Manpower. Division of Nursing 1.53, 4.27-.30
U.S. Bureau of Health Planning and Resources Development 1.30, 1.54
U.S. Bureau of Health Resources Development 4.31-.32
U.S. Bureau of Labor Statistics 1.55, 3.46
U.S. Bureau of Radiological Health 5.9
U.S. Bureau of the Census 1.38, 1.56, 1.88, 1.106, 2.4, 2.5, 7.1-.10
U.S. Center for Disease Control 2.6, 3.12, 3.1-.2, 3.48, 3.50-.54, 5.10-.11
U.S. Center for Disease Control. Nutrition Program 3.43
U.S. Commission for the Control of Epilepsy and Its Consequences 3.38
U.S. Congress. Congressional Budget Office 1.107, 6.20
U.S. Congress. House of Representatives. Committee on Interstate and Foreign Commerce 1.31
U.S. Congress. House of Representatives. Committee on Ways and Means 1.108
U.S. Council on Wage and Price Stability 6.21
U.S. Department of Commerce 1.109
U.S. Department of Health, Education, and Welfare 1.20, 1.39
U.S. Department of Labor. Bureau of Labor Statistics 7.11-.13
U.S. Division of Health Manpower Intelligence 4.33
U.S. Food and Drug Administration. National Clearinghouse for Poison Control Centers 3.9
U.S. Health Resources Administration 1.40, 1.110-.111, 4.3, 4.34
U.S. Health Services and Mental Health Administration 6.22
U.S. Indian Health Service 2.7, 3.58
U.S. Indian Health Service. Office of Program Statistics 5.12
U.S. National Cancer Institute 3.18-.20
U.S. National Cancer Institute. Biometry Branch 3.21-.22, 6.23
U.S. National Cancer Institute. End Results Section 3.23-.24
U.S. National Center for Education Statistics 4.50-.51
U.S. National Center for Health Statistics 1.41, 1.57, 1.71, 1.89, 1.112, 2.8-.14, 3.3-.4, 3.44-.45, 4.35-.38, 4.4-.7, 5.13, 5.16
U.S. National Clearinghouse for Smoking and Health 3.49
U.S. National Clearinghouse on Aging 1.113
U.S. National Clearinghouse on Alcohol Information 1.58
U.S. National Commission on Diabetes 3.26
U.S. National Criminal Justice Information and Statistics Service 7.14
U.S. National Health Survey 1.90-.93
U.S. National Heart and Lung Institute 2.15, 3.39-.40

Author Index

U.S. National Institute for Occupational Safety and Health 2.16, 3.47
U.S. National Institute of Arthritis, Metabolism and Digestive Diseases 3.27
U.S. National Institute of Health. Nephrology Cost Group 6.25
U.S. National Institute of Mental Health 3.41-.42, 4.8, 5.17
U.S. National Institute of Neurological and Communicative Disorders and Stroke 4.39, 6.24
U.S. National Institute on Aging 1.114
U.S. National Institute on Alcohol Abuse and Alcoholism 3.11
U.S. National Institute on Drug Abuse 3.30-.37
U.S. National Library of Medicine 1.58A
U.S. Office of Management and Budget 1.21-.22
U.S. Office of the Federal Register 1.23
U.S. Public Health Service. Federal Security Agency 3.59
U.S. Public Health Service. Office of International Health 1.115
U.S. Social Security Administration 1.42, 3.28-.29, 5.18-.20
U.S. Social Security Administration. Office of Research and Statistics 6.26-.31, 7.15
U.S. Veterans Administration 3.60
Urban and Rural Systems Associates 4.40

W

Wasserman, Paul 1.24-.25
Waterhouse, J. 3.25
Weise, Frieda (O.) 1.59
Wilner, Daniel M. 1.15
World Health Organization 1.116-.17, 3.5
Worthington, Nancy L. 6.9
Wright, Nancy D. 1.26

Y

Yakes, Nancy 1.17

Z

Zeisset, Paul T. 1.72, 1.76

TITLE INDEX

This index includes all titles of books, reports, and proceedings cited in the text. In some cases titles have been shortened. References are to entry numbers and alphabetization is letter by letter.

A

Abortion Surveillance 5.10
Abstracts of Health Care Management Studies 1.60
Abstracts of Hospital Management Studies 1.60
Accident Facts 3.8
Adult Use of Tobacco--1975 3.49
American Statistics Index 1.61
Analysis of Doctor's Degrees Awarded to Men and Women 1970-71 through 1974-75 4.50
Analytical and Special Study Reports 3.41
Analytical Studies, 1964-- 1.89
Annotated Bibliography of Health Economics, An 1.45
Annotated Bibliography of Publications, An 1.52
Annual Report on Dental Education 4.41
Area Resource File 1.74
ASI 1.81
Atlas of Cancer Mortality among U.S. Nonwhites, 1950-69 3.18
Atlas of Cancer Mortality for U.S. Counties, 1950-1969 3.19

B

Basic Statistics for Health Science Students 1.13

Bibliographic Guide to Statistics and Health Planning Information 1.59
Bibliography of the Socioeconomic Aspects of Medicine 1.44
Bibliography on Health Indexes 1.62
Birth, Stillbirth, and Infant Mortality Statistics, 1915-1936 2.4
Black Americans, a Chartbook, Bulletin 1699 7.11
BLS Data Bank Files and Statistical Routines 1.75
Botulism in the United States, 1899-1973 3.12
Bureau of the Census Catalog 1.33
Bureau of the Census Catalog of Publications, 1790-1972 1.38

C

Cancer Facts and Figures 3.13
Cancer Incidence in Five Continents (Doll) 3.15
Cancer Incidence in Five Continents (Waterhouse) 3.25
Cancer Patient Survival 3.23
Cancer Rates and Risks 3.21
Catalogue of Publications, 1962-71 1.41
CATLINE 1.82
Changes in the Costs of Treatment of Selected Illnesses, 1951-1964-1971 6.19

Title Index

Characteristics of Black Physicians in the U.S. 4.31
Chartbook on Smoking, Tobacco, and Health 3.48
Checklist of State Publications 1.34
Comparative Statistics on Health Facilities and Population 3.1
Compendium of National Health Expenditures Data 6.7
Conference Or Committee Reports and Analytical Review of Literature 3.41
Congressional District Data Book 7.1
Contraceptive Services for Adolescents 5.1
Costs of Education in the Health Professions 6.13
County and City Data Book, 1977 7.2
Current Listings and Topical Index to the Vital and Health Statistics Series, 1962-77 1.71
Current Population Reports, Federal-State Cooperative Program for Population Estimates 7.3
Current Population Reports, Population Characteristics 7.4
Current Population Reports, Population Estimates and Projections 7.5

D

Data Acquisition and Analysis Handbook for Health Planners 1.29
Data Evaluation and Methods Research, 1963-- 1.89
Data for Health Planning 1.51
Data from the Client Oriented Data Acquisition Process (CODAP), Series E 3.30
Data from the Health Examination Survey 1.89, 3.3
Data from the Health Interview Survey 3.4
Data from the Health Interview Survey 1963-- 1.89
Data from the Health Records Survey, no. 1-24, 1965-74 1.89
Data from the National Drug Abuse Treatment Utilization Survey (NDATUS), Series F 3.31
Data from the National Natality and Mortality Surveys, no. 1-15, 1961-76 1.89
Data from the National Survey of Family Growth, 1977-- 1.89
Data on Health Resources 1.89, 4.4, 4.35
Data on Health Resources Utilization 1.89, 5.13
Data on Mortality 1.89, 2.8
Data on Natality, Marriage and Divorce 1.89, 2.9
Deaf Population of the United States, The 3.56
Decennial Census Data for Selected Health Occupations 4.36
Demographic Yearbook 1.104
Determinants of Expenditures for Physicians' Services in the United States, 1948-1968 6.22
Diabetes Data 3.27
Dictionary of Statistical Terms, A 1.28
Directory of Computerized Data Files, Software, and Related Technical Reports, A 1.80
Directory of Data Sources on Racial and Ethnic Minorities 1.55
Directory of Federal Statistics for Local Areas 1.56
Directory of Government Document Collections and Librarians 1.16
Directory of Nursing Home Facilities 4.3
Directory of On-going Research on Cancer Epidemiology 1.18
Directory of Online Information Resources 1.73
Disability Survey 71 3.28
Disability Survey 72 3.29
Discharge Summary 5.12
Discursive Dictionary of Health Care, A 1.31
Distribution of Dentists in the United States by State, Region, District and County, 1976 4.11
Distribution of Health Personnel 1.49
Documents and Committee Reports 1.89
Drug Use among American High School Students 3.32

Title Index

E

Earnings Distribution in the United States, 1969 7.15
Economic Cost of Alcohol Abuse, The 6.6
Encyclopedia of Associations 1.17
Epidemiology of Aging 1.114
Epidemiology of Cancer in Texas 3.16
Estimates of the Fraction of Cancer in the United States Related to Occupational Diseases 3.14
Estimating the Cost of Illness 6.17
Eurohealth Handbook 1.97
EXCERPTA MEDICA 1.83
Excerpta Medica, Section 17 1.63
Excerpta Medica, Section 36 1.64
Exploratory Study of Women in the Health Professions Schools 4.40

F

Facts about Nursing 4.14
Federal Health Dollar, The 6.14
Federal Statistical Directory 1.21
Foundations of Epidemiology 1.11
Framingham Study, The 3.39

G

Guide to Data for Health Systems Planners 1.54
Guide to the Collection and Use of Health Expenditures and Utilization Data for Health Planning Agencies 1.30
Guide to the Health Care Field 4.2
Guide to U.S. Government Statistics 1.32

H

Handbook of Community Health 1.7
Handbook of Labor Statistics 7.12
HAS-MAP 1.80b
HAS-MONITREND 1.80a
HEALTH 1.84
Health: United States 1.110
Health and Medical Economics 1.43
Health and Work in America 3.47
Health Differentials between White and Nonwhite Americans 1.107

Health Insurance for the Aged 5.18
Health Insurance Notes 5.19
Health in the Later Years of Life--Selected Data from the National Center for Health Statistics 1.112
Health Manpower. A County and Metropolitan Area Data Book 4.37
Health of the Disadvantaged 1.111
Health Organizations of the United States, Canada, and Internationally 1.24
Health Planning 1.65
Health Planning: Weekly Government Abstract 1.65
Health Planning and Administration 1.84
Health Professions Schools 4.47
Health Resources Statistics 4.5, 4.38
Health Services R & D Data Tapes 1.78
Health Service Use--National Trends and Variations, 1953-1971 5.4
Health Statistics: A Manual for Teachers of Medical Students 1.12
Health Statistics Plan 1.20
Health Statistics Series A 1.90
Health Statistics Series B 1.91
Health Statistics Series C 1.92
Health Statistics Series D 1.93
Health Status of Children 3.57a
Hemodialysis Costs in the U.S. 6.25
Heroin Indicators Trend Report 3.33
Historical Statistics of the United States 1.106
Hospital Literature Index 1.66
Hospitals: A County and Metropolitan Area Data Book 4.6
Hospital Statistics 5.2

I

Illness among Indians, 1965-69 3.58
Illness and Medical Care among 2,500,000 Persons in 83 Cities with Special Reference to Socio-Economic Factors 3.59
Improvement in Infant and Perinatal Mortality in the United States, 1965-1973 2.3

Title Index

Index Medicus 1.67
Index to 1970 Census Summary Tapes 1.76
Index to Selected 1970 Census Reports 1.72
Indian Health Trends and Services 2.7
Institutional Characteristics of U.S. Medical Schools, 1975-1976, Final Report 4.48
Interagency Conference on Nursing Statistics 1.53
International Health Costs and Expenditures 6.12
Interpretation and Uses of Medical Statistics 1.3
Introduction to Epidemiology, An 1.1
Introduction to Medical Statistics, An 1.10
Introduction to Public Health 1.15
Introductory Biostatistics for Health Sciences 1.5

K

Killers and Cripplers, The 1.98, 3.57

L

Length of Stay by Diagnosis 5.20
Length of Stay in PAS Hospitals, by Diagnosis 5.5
Leukemias and Lymphomas 3.17
Life Insurance Fact Book 6.1
Lilly Digest 6.14a
Long-term Care: Actual Cost Estimates 6.20

M

Management Effectiveness Measures for NIDA Drug Abuse Treatment Programs, Final Report 6.18
Marihuana and Health 3.34
Measurement of Expenditures for Outpatient Physician and Dental Services, The 6.15
Medical and Health Information Directory 1.19
Medical Care Chart Book 1.96
Medical Care Costs and Prices 6.26
Medical Care Use by a Group of Fully Insured Aged 5.8

Medical Education in the United States 4.42
Medical Risks 1.100
Medical Socioeconomic Research Sources (MEDSOC) 1.68
MEDLINE 1.85
MEDOC 1.86
MEDOC: A Computerized Index to U.S. Government Documents in the Medical and Health Sciences 1.69
Mental Health Facilities Reports 3.41, 4.8, 5.17
Methodology Reports 3.41
Minorities and Women in the Health Fields 4.9
Minority Health Chart Book 1.95
Minority Student Opportunities in the United States Medical Schools, 1975-76 4.43
MMWR: Morbidity and Mortality Weekly Report 2.6, 3.1
Monthly Vital Statistics Report 2.10
Mortality Statistics, 1900-1936 2.5
Most Frequently Occurring Diagnoses in VA Hospitals, 1971-1976 3.60

N

National Directory of State Agencies, 1976-77, The 1.26
National Estimates of Faculty Manpower in U.S. Medical Schools, Final Report 4.45
National Halothane Study, The 3.6
National Health Directory 1.19a
National Health Insurance Resource Book 1.108
National Library of Medicine Current Catalog 1.58a
National Prescription Audit, Company Report 5.5a
National Prescription Audit, National Hospital Survey 5.5b
National Prescription Audit, Therapeutic Category Report 5.5c
National Reporting System for Family Planning Services 5.14
National Survey of Drug Abuse 3.35
Nation's Psychiatrists--1970 Survey, The 4.15
Nation's Use of Health Resources, The 5.15

Title Index

Neiss News 3.7
Neurological and Communicative Disorders 6.24
NINCDS Manpower Surveys 4.39
1975 Fee Survey 6.2
1977 Survey of Dental Practice 6.3
Nonmedical Use of Psychoactive Substance 3.36
NTIS 1.87
Nurses Almanac, The 1.99A
Nursing Homes—a County and Metropolitan Area Data Book 4.7
Nursing Personnel in Hospitals: 1970 Survey of Hospitals Registered with the American Hospital Association 4.27
Nursing Personnel in Hospitals: 1972 Public Health Survey 4.28
Nursing Personnel in Hospitals Registered with AHA 4.32

O

Occupational Injuries and Illnesses in the United States, by Industry 3.46
Occupational Mortality in Washington State, 1950-1971 2.16
Optometric Manpower Resources, 1973 4.20
Osteopathic Physicians in the United States 4.10

P

Participation of Women and Minorities on U.S. Medical School Faculties 4.18
Patterns of Dental Services Utilization in the United States 5.6
Personal Health Care Expenditures by State 6.9
Physician Distribution and Medical Licensure in the United States 4.12
Physicians for the Future 4.44
Plan for Nationwide Action on Epilepsy 3.38
Poison Control Statistics 3.9
Population Exposure to X-Rays, U.S. 1970 5.9
Population Index 1.70

Practical Epidemiology 1.2
Preliminary Findings of the First Health and Nutrition Examination Survey, United States, 1971-72: Anthropometric and Clinical Findings 3.44
Preliminary Findings of the First Health and Nutrition Examination Survey, United States, 1971-72: Dietary Intake and Biochemical Findings 3.45
Prescription Drug Data Summary 6.27
Prescription Drug Industry Factbook 6.16
Preventive Medicine and Public Health 1.14
Primer of Epidemiology 1.6
Proceedings of the International Conference on Women in Health, June 16-18, 1975, Washington, D.C. 4.21
Program and Collection Procedures 1.89
Public and High Blood Pressure, The 3.40
Publications Catalog 1.39
Public Health and Community Medicine for the Allied Medical Professions 1.4

R

Reference Data on Socioeconomic Issues of Health 1.99, 6.4
Reference Data on the Profile of Medical Practice 1.94, 4.13, 5.3, 6.5
Registered Pharmacists in (state), 1973 4.33
Report of the National Commission on Diabetes to the Congress of the United States 3.26
Report Series on Mental Health Statistics 3.41
Report to the Congress on the Status of Health Professions Personnel in the United States 4.26
Research and Statistics Note 6.28
RN's One and Five Years after Graduation 4.19

Title Index

S

Selected National Data Sources for Health Planners 1.50
Selected Publications on Statistics and Demographic Research on Alcohol Use and Abuse 1.58
Sexually Transmitted Disease (STD) Statistical Letter 3.53
Short Textbook of Medical Statistics, A 1.8
Size and Shape of the Medical Care Dollar 6.29
Smoking and General Mortality among U.S. Veterans, 1954-1959 2.15
Social Indicators, 1976 1.109
Social Security Bulletin 6.30
Some Statistics on Baccalaureate and Higher Degree Programs in Nursing 1975-76 4.46
Sourcebook: Nursing Personnel 4.17
Sourcebook of Criminal Justice Statistics 7.14
Sourcebook of Health Insurance Data 6.11
STD Fact Sheet 3.54
Standardized Micro-Data Tape Transcripts 1.79
Standard Medical Almanac 1.101
State Estimates of Disability and Utilization of Medical Services 5.16
Statistical Abstract of the United States 1.102
Statistical Notes 3.42
Statistical Portrait of Women in the United States, A 7.6
Statistical Principles in Health Care Information 1.9
Statistical Profile of Hospital Outpatient Services in the U.S., A 5.7
Statistical Reports on Older Americans 1.113
Statistical Services of the United States Government 1.22
Statistical Yearbook 1.105
Statistics on Blindness in the Model Reporting Area, 1968-70 3.55
Statistics on Consumption of Alcohol and Alcoholism 3.10
Statistics Sources 1.25

Study of Participation of Women in the Health Care Industry Labor Force 4.34
Study of Physicians' Fees, A 6.21
Study of Physicians' Income in the Pre-Medicare Period, 1965 6.31
Summary Tape Processing Centers 1.77
Supply, Need, and Distribution of Anesthesiologists and Nurse Anesthetists in the U.S., 1972 and 1980 4.22
Supply and Availability of Physician Services, The 4.16
Supply of Health Manpower, The 4.23
Surgery in the United States 1.103
Surveillance Reports 3.2
Survey of Foreign Nurse Graduates 4.29
Survey of Registered Nurses Employed in Physicians Offices, September 1973 4.30
Survey of Selected Hospital Manpower, February 1973, Preliminary Report 4.24
Syncrisis 1.115

T

Ten-State Nutrition Survey, 1968-1970 3.43
Third National Cancer Survey 6.23
Third National Cancer Survey--Advanced Three-Year Report, 1969-71 Incidence 3.22
Third Special Report to the U.S. Congress on Alcohol and Health 3.11
Treatment and Survival Patterns for Black and White Cancer Patients, 1955-1964 3.24
Tuberculosis in the United States 3.50
Tuberculosis in the World 3.51
Tuberculosis Statistics 3.52

U

U.S. Cancer Mortality by County, 1950-69 3.20
U.S. Census of Population-1(5) 7.8

Title Index

U.S. Census of Population-1970: Employment Profiles of Selected Low-Income Areas, Final Report 7.9
U.S. Census of Population, 1970: Volume II, Subject Reports 7.10
United States Decennial Life Tables for 1969-71, Vol. II, Nos. 1-51 2.11
United States Government Manual 1.23
United States Immunization Survey 5.11
United States Life Tables, 1969-71 2.12
U.S. Working Woman 7.13
Urban Atlas 7.7

V

Vital and Health Statistics Series 1.89
Vital Statistics--Special Reports 1.88
Vital Statistics Advance Data 2.13
Vital Statistics of the United States 2.14
Vital Statistics Rates in the United States, 1900-1940 2.2
Vital Statistics Rates in the United States, 1940-60 2.1

W

Weekly Epidemiological Record 3.5
Women in Health Careers 4.25
Women's Participation in First-Professional Degree Programs in Medicine, and Law, 1969-70 through 1974-75 4.51
World Health Statistics Annual 1.116
World Health Statistics Report 1.117

Y

Young Men and Drugs 3.37

SUBJECT INDEX

References are to entry numbers and underlined numbers refer to main subject areas within the text. Alphabetization is letter by letter.

A

Abortion
  legal 5.10
  statistical series on 3.2
Accidents and injuries 3.6-.9, 3.59
  alcohol and traffic 3.11
  death from 2.14
  economic costs of 6.8
  indexes and abstracts on 1.63
  of Indians 5.12
  occupational 3.46
  statistical series on 1.89
Adolescent Health in Harlem (survey) 3.57
Adolescents, contraception services for 5.1
Africa, cancer incidence in 3.25
Age, statistics on. See Population and demographic characteristics
Aged. See Geriatrics
Alabama
  health statistic sources of B.1
  regional depository libraries of D.1-.2
Alaska, health statistic sources of B.2
Alcohol and alcoholism 3.10-.11
  bibliography on 1.58
  consumption of 3.10
  economic costs of 6.6

journals on A.23
  students and 3.32
  young men and 3.37
Allergies 1.98
Allied health personnel
  education of 4.42
  in the field of nursing 4.14
  manpower studies of 4.23-.24
  statistical series on 1.116
  women and minorities as 4.9
  See also Physician's assistants
Ambulatory care 5.7, 5.13
  bibliography on 1.54
  facilities for 4.4-.5
  measurement of expenditures for 6.15
  statistical series on 1.89
American Association of Medical Colleges 4.45
American Burn Association C.1
American Cancer Society C.2
American College of Surgeons C.3
American Dental Association C.4
American Diabetes Association C.5
American Heart Association C.6
American Hospital Association 4.32, C.7
  data files compiled by 1.80 a, 1.84
American Indians
  cancer among 3.18
  illness among 3.58
  inpatient data on 5.12
  vital and health statistics for 2.7

Subject Index

American Nurses' Association 4.29, C.8
Anesthesiologists, distribution and supply of 4.22
Appendicitis, cost changes in the treatment of 6.19
Area Health Education Centers (AHEC), directory for 1.19
Area Resources File, guide to 1.74
Arizona
    health statistic sources of B.4
    regional depository libraries of D.3-.4
Arkansas, health statistic sources of B.5
Arthritis, statistical series on 1.98
Arthritis Foundation C.9
Asbestos, cancer and 3.14
Aseptic meningitis. See Meningitis, aseptic
Asia, cancer incidence in 3.25
Association of American Medical Colleges C.10
Audiology, manpower studies in 4.39
Australia, cancer incidence in 3.25
Automobile accidents. See Accidents and injuries
Auxiliary health personnel. See Allied health personnel

B

Belgium, health care costs in 6.12
Bibliographic Retrieval Services (company), data files of 1.85, 1.86, 1.87, E.1
Birth control. See Contraception; Family planning
Birth statistics. See Natality
Black lung disease, social security programs for 6.30
Blacks 7.11
    cancer among 3.18, 3.24
    health status of 1.95, 1.107, 1.111
    as physicans 4.31
    See also Adolescent Health in Harlem (survey)
Blindness. See Vision and hearing
Blood disorders, economic costs of 6.8
Blood pressure. See Hypertension

Blue Cross Association C.11
    journals published by A.9
Botulism 3.12
    statistical series on 3.2
Breast cancer, cost changes in the treatment of 6.19
Brucellosis, statistical series on 3.2

C

California
    health statistic sources of B.6
    guides to 1.47
    regional depository library of D.5
Canada, health care costs in 6.12
Cancer 3.13-.25
    among non-whites 3.16, 3.18
    directory of research on 1.18
    hospital payments by patients having 6.23
    journals on A.21
    mortality rates for 3.18-.20
    occupational related 3.14
    statistical series on 1.98
    See also Breast cancer; types of cancer (e.g., Hodgkin's disease)
Census 7.8-.10
    catalogs and indexes relating to 1.33, 1.38, 1.72, 1.76-.77
    collection and procedure data on 1.15
Cerebral palsy, statistical series on 1.98
Chemicals, associated with cancer 3.14
Childbearing
    economic costs of 6.8
    statistical series on 1.89
Children
    diseases of 3.59
    health status of 3.57a
    See also Infants
Chinese Americans, cancer among 3.18
Chronic disease and illness 3.57, 3.59
    among children 3.57a

Subject Index

bibliography on 1.57
indexes and abstracts on 1.60
journals on A.18
statistical series on 1.112, 3.3
Circulatory diseases, economic costs of 6.8
Cocaine. See Drug abuse
College students. See Medical students
Colorado
  health statistic sources of B.7
  regional depository library of D.6
Coma 3.26
Commission on Professional and Hospital Activities C.12
  data file compiled by 1.80b
  Professional Activity Study 5.5
Committee to Combat Huntington's Disease C.13
Communicable disease. See Infectious disease
Community medicine. See Public health
Community mental health centers 3.42
Congenital malformations
  economic costs of 6.8
  statistical series on 3.2
Connecticut
  health statistic sources of B.8
  regional depository library of D.7
Contraception, for adolescents 5.1.
  See also Family planning
Coronary heart disease 3.26

D

Data bases. See Machine-readable files
Deafness. See Vision and hearing
Death. See Mortality
Delaware, health statistic sources of B.9
Demographic statistics. See Population and demographic characteristics
Denmark, health care costs in 6.12
Dental care 5.4
  among children 3.57a
  measurement of expenditures for 6.13
  statistical series on 1.89
  utilization patterns in 5.6

Dental education 4.41, 4.47
  costs of 6.12
Dentistry
  minorities in 4.9
  women in 4.9, 4.11, 4.34, 4.40
Dentists
  fees of 6.2-.3, 6.26
  manpower studies of 4.11, 4.23, 4.38
  statistical series on 1.89
Developing Countries 1.115
Diabetes 3.26-.27
  journals on A.10
Diagnostic medicine, in veterans hospitals 3.60
Digestive disorders
  economic costs of 6.8
  statistical series on 1.98
Diphtheria, statistical series on 3.2
  immunization data of 5.11
Disability 3.28-.29, 5.4, 5.16
  bibliography on 1.54
  economic costs of 6.17
  statistical series on 1.89, 1.98, 1.109, 1.112, 3.4
Disease
  alcohol related 3.11
  bibliography on 1.43
  children and 3.59
  costs of 1.115, 6.8
  statistical series on 1.98, 1.99A, 1.101
  See also Chronic disease; Foodborne disease; Infectious disease; Occupational health and diseases; Waterborne disease; names of diseases (e.g., Heart disease)

District of Columbia. See Washington, D.C.
Divorce 2.9-.10
  statistical series on 1.89, 1.104
Doctors. See Physicians
Drug abuse 3.30-.37, 7.14
  cost/benefit analysis in the treatment of 6.18
Drugs. See Pharmaceuticals
Duodenal ulcer. See Ulcers, duodenal

Subject Index

E

Elderly. See Geriatrics
Encephalitis, statistical series on 3.2
Endocrine diseases, economic costs of 6.8
England. See Great Britain
Enterovirus disease, statistical series on 3.2
Environmental health, journals on A.8
Epidemiology
    dictionaries on 1.31
    journals on A.5, A.16
    statistical series on 1.116, 3.5
    textbooks on 1.1-.2, 1.4, 1.6-.7, 1.9, 1.11, 1.14-.15
    See also names of diseases (e.g., Measles)
Epilepsy 3.38
    statistical series on 1.98
Epilepsy Foundation of America C.14
Eskimos, illness among 3.58
Ethnic groups. See Minority groups; names of minority groups (e.g., Blacks)
Europe, cancer incidence in 3.25
Europe, Western, health care statistics of 1.97

F

Family planning, statistical series on 1.89, 5.13-.14. See also Contraception
Family practitioners, distribution and supply of 4.16
Federal government
    directories to agencies of 1.19, 1.21-.23, B.56-.98
    guide to the statistics of 1.32, 1.36, 1.46-.47, 1.56-.57, 1.61, 1.80
    health care expenditures by 6.13
    role of in health 1.101
Fertility rates 2.14, 3.59, 7.6
    indexes and abstracts on 1.70
    statistical series on 1.89
    textbooks on 1.10
Fetus, mortality of 1.104, 2.3-.4, 2.14

Florida
    health statistic sources of B.11
    regional depository library of D.8
Food and Agriculture Organization, bibliography of the publications of 1.35
Foodborne disease, statistical series on 3.2. See also Botulism
Fractures, cost changes in the treatment of 6.19
France, health care costs in 6.12

G

General practitioners. See Family practitioners
Genetic diseases, statistical series on 1.98
Genitourinary diseases, economic costs of 6.8
Georgia
    health statistic sources of B.12
    regional depository library of D.9
Geriatrics
    statistical series on 1.99A, 1.112-14
    utilization studies in 5.8
    See also Medicare
Germany, West, health care costs in 6.12
Government. See Federal government; State government
Government documents, library collections of 1.16, D.1-.45
Guam, health statistic sources of B.13

H

Hallucinogens. See Drug abuse
Halothane anesthesia, postoperative hepatitis with 3.6
Handicapped, statistical series on 1.99A. See also Mental health and illness
Harlem. See Adolescent Health in Harlem (survey)

Subject Index

Hawaii
 health statistic sources of B.14
 regional depository library of D.10
Health care 3.59
 guides to machine readable files on
  1.80
 indexing and abstracting services on
  1.66, 1.68
 journals on A.15, A.24
 statistical series on 1.89, 1.96,
  1.106, 1.108-.109
Health care costs and expenditures
  4.14, 6.1-.31
 bibliographies on 1.43, 1.45,
  1.50
 for cancer 6.23
 for diabetes 3.26
 dictionaries and handbooks on
  1.30
 for the disabled 3.29
 for drug abuse treatment 3.31
 for epilepsy treatment 3.38
 for hemodialysis 6.25
 indexes and abstracts on 1.60,
  1.65-.66, 1.68
 journals on A.15, A.25, A.32
 for neurological and sensory disorders 6.24
 statistical series on 1.96, 1.99-
  .99A, 1.101, 1.103, 1.117
 minority groups 1.111
 Western European 1.97
 by state 6.9
Health care planning
 bibliographies on 1.50-.51,
  1.54, 1.59
 dictionaries and handbooks on
  1.27, 1.29-.31
 indexing and abstracting services
  on 1.65, 1.84, 1.87
 newsletters and journals on A.3,
  A.12
Health education. See Medical
  education
Health facilities 4.1-.8, 4.12,
  4.14, 4.37, 5.2
 bibliographies on 1.50, 1.54
 cost of patient care in 6.23,
  6.26, 6.28-.29
 data files on 1.80a

drug purchases by 5.5b
federal expenditures for construction of 6.14
indexes and abstracting services
  on 1.60, 1.65, 1.71
journals on A.14, A.27
length of stay in 5.5
manpower studies in 4.24
for mental health 4.8, 5.17
nurses and nursing in 4.27-.28,
  4.32
population and 4.1
statistical series on 1.89, 1.96,
  1.99A, 1.101, 1.108,
  1.116-.117
West European 1.97
for tuberculosis 3.52
use of by Medicare patients
  5.18, 5.20
See also Home care; Medical
  records; Nursing homes;
  Veterans hospitals
Health insurance. See Insurance,
  health
Health Insurance Institute C.15
Health manpower 4.4-.5, 4.9-.40
 bibliographies on 1.49, 1.52,
  1.57
 dictionaries on 1.31
 federal expenditures for training
  in 6.14
 in hospitals 4.24
 indexes and abstracts on 1.60,
  1.65-.68, 1.71
 minorities and 4.9
 statistical series on 1.89, 1.96,
  1.101, 1.103, 1.108,
  1.116-.117
 minority groups 1.111
 West European 1.97
 women and 4.9, 4.21, 4.25,
  4.34
 See also Allied health personnel;
  Dentists; Medical specialties;
  Nurses and nursing; Physicians
Health services utilization 4.14,
  5.1-.20
 the aged and 5.8
 bibliography on 1.57

Subject Index

in dental care 5.6
dictionaries and handbooks on 1.29-.30
in drug abuse treatment 3.31
indexes and abstracts on 1.60, 1.65-.68
by Indians 5.12
by Medicare patients 5.18-.20
statistical series on 1.89, 1.94, 1.103, 1.112, 3.4
  minority groups 1.95, 1.107, 1.111
See also Medical records
Health statistics
  associations providing C.1-.30
  collection, interpretation, and use of 1.3, 1.8-.10, 1.12-.13, 1.89
  general references on 1.1-.117
    bibliographies 1.43-.59
    catalogs 1.32-.42
    dictionaries and handbooks 1.27-.31
    directories 1.16-.26
    indexes and abstracts 1.60-.72
    machine readable files 1.73-.87
    textbooks 1.1-.15
    vital and health statistics series 1.88-.117
  government agencies providing B.1-.98
  international agencies providing B.99-.102
  newsletters and journals on A.1-.32
  regional depository libraries containing D.1-.45
  suppliers of bibliographic data files for E.1-.4
  See also Accidents and injuries; Disease; Illness; Morbidity; Mortality; Natality; Population and demographic characteristics; Vital statistics; headings beginning with the terms "Health" (e.g., Health care) and "Medical" (e.g., Medical education); specific diseases (e.g., Cancer)

Health Systems Agencies (HSA), directories to 1.19-.19a
Heart disease 3.39. See also Coronary heart disease
Hemodialysis, costs of performing 6.25
Hepatitis
  drug abuse and 3.33
  postoperative 3.6
  statistical series on 3.2
Heroin. See Drug abuse
High blood pressure. See Hypertension
Hodgkin's disease 3.17
Holland. See Netherlands
Home care
  bibliography on 1.54
  statistical series on 1.112
Hospital Administrative Services, data files compiled by 1.80a
Hospitals. See Health facilities; Psychiatric hospitals; Veterans hospitals
Hypertension 3.40
  statistical series on 1.98

I

Idaho
  health statistic sources of B.15
  regional depository library of D.11
Illinois
  health statistic sources of B.16
    bibliographical guide to 1.59
  regional depository library of D.12
Illness 3.59
  among Indians and Eskimos 3.58
  economic costs of 6.8, 6.17
  statistical series on 1.89
  See also Chronic disease and illness; Disease
Indiana
  health statistic sources of B.17
  regional depository library of D.13
Indians. See American Indians
Industrial health and diseases. See

Subject Index

Occupational health and diseases
Infants, mortality among 1.104, 2.3-.4, 2.14
Infectious disease
  epidemiology of 1.14
  journals on A.19
  statistical series on 1.98, 1.116-.117, 3.2, 3.5
  See also names of infectious diseases (e.g., Mumps)
Infectious Disease Society of America C.16
Influenza, statistical series on 3.2
  immunization data in 5.11
Insurance, dictionaries on 1.31
Insurance, health 6.11
  benefit payments of 6.1
  expenditures of private programs for 6.7
  indexes and abstracts on 1.66
  statistical series on 1.96, 1.108
  See also Medicaid; Medicare
Insurance, social 6.28, 6.30
  journals on A.30
International Agency for Research on Cancer (IARC) B.99
International Association of Boards of Examiners in Optometry 4.20
International Conference on Women in Health (1975), proceedings of 4.21
Iowa
  health statistic sources of B.18
  regional depository library of D.14

J

Japanese-Americans, cancer among 3.18

K

Kansas
  health statistic sources of B.19
  regional depository library of D.15
Kentucky
  health statistic sources of B.20
  regional depository library of D.16

L

Leptospirosis, statistical series on 3.2
Leukemia 3.17
Life expectancy
  statistical series on 1.109, 1.112, 1.114
  of women 7.6
Lockheed Information Systems, data files of 1.87, E.2
Louisiana
  health statistic sources of B.21
  regional depository library of D.17
Low-income groups, child health among 3.57a
LSD. See Drug abuse
Lymphosarcoma 3.17

M

Machine-readable files
  bibliographic files 1.81-.87
  data files 1.80a-.80b
  guides to 1.73-.80
Maine
  health statistic sources of B.22
  regional depository library of D.18
Malaria, statistical series on 3.2
Marihuana. See Drug abuse
Marriage 2.9-.10
  statistical series on 1.89, 1.104
Maryland
  health statistic sources of .23
  regional depository library of D.19
Massachusetts
  health statistic sources of B.24
  regional depository library of D.20
Measles, statistical series on 3.2
  immunization data of 5.11
Medicaid
  dictionaries on 1.31
  directory of officials in 1.19a
  utilization of by state 5.4
Medical and health organizations, associations, and agencies, directories to 1.17, 1.19, 1.24
Medical care. See Health care
Medical education 4.41-.51

Subject Index

costs of 6.13
faculty manpower studies in 4.45
  on women and minorities 4.18
indexes and abstracts on 1.65
journals on A.20
minorities as students in 4.43
statistical series on 1.101-.102
women as students in 4.25, 4.51
Medical literature and Analysis
  Retrieval System (MEDLARS)
  1.58a, 1.82, 1.84
Medical records, data files created
  from 1.80b
Medical research
  on epilepsy 3.38
  federal expenditures for 6.14
Medical specialties
  manpower studies of 4.16, 4.23
  statistical series on 1.116
  women in 4.25
  See also names of medical special-
    ties (e.g. Podiatry)
Medical statistics. See Health
  statistics
Medicare 5.18-.20
  dictionaries on 1.31
  directory of officials in 1.19a
  impact on physician income 6.31
Medicines. See Pharmaceuticals
MEDLARS. See Medical Literature
  Analysis and Retrieval System
  (MEDLARS)
MEDLINE 1.85
  directory of centers for 1.19
  indexes and abstracts to 1.67
Meningitis, aseptic, statistical series
  on 3.2
Mental health and illness 3.41-.42,
  5.17
  economic costs of 6.8
  facilities for 4.8
  of Indians 5.12
  statistical series on 1.98
  See also Handicapped; Psychiatric
    hospitals; Psychiatrists
Metabolic diseases, economic costs
  of 6.8
Methadone, cost/benefit analysis of
  the use of 6.18

Michigan
  health statistic sources of B.25
  regional depository libraries of
    D.21-.22
Migration 7.2
  of blacks 7.11
  international 1.104
  of women 7.6
Minnesota
  health statistic sources of B.26
  regional depository library of
    D.23
Minority groups
  bibliography on 1.55
  cancer among 3.16, 3.18, 3.23
  child health among 3.57a
  in the health professions 4.9
  on medical faculties 4.18
  as medical students 4.43
  statistical series on 1.95, 1.99A,
    1.107, 1.111
Mississippi
  health statistic sources of B.27
  regional depository library of
    D.24
Missouri, health statistic sources of
  B.28
Montana
  health statistic sources of B.29
  regional depository library of
    D.25
Morbidity rates 2.6
  bibliography on 1.54
  for diabetes 3.27
  economic costs associated with
    6.17
  indexes and abstracts on 1.63,
    1.68
  for Indians 5.12
  statistical series on 1.88, 1.96,
    1.99, 1.116, 3.1-.5
    developing countries
      1.115
    West European 1.97
  textbooks on 1.1, 1.10
  trends of 6.10
  for tuberculosis 3.50-.51
Mortality 2.1-.6, 2.8, 2.10,
  2.14
  accidental 3.8

Subject Index

cancer and 3.13, 3.17-.21
diabetes and 3.27
economic costs associated with 6.17
epilepsy and 3.38
heroin and 3.33
indexes and abstracts on 1.63, 1.67-.68, 1.70
from neurological and sensory disorders 6.24
occupational related 2.16
postoperative 3.6
statistical series on 1.89, 1.96, 1.99, 1.100, 1.104, 1.112, 1.114, 3.1-.2, 7.2
    underdeveloped countries 1.115
    West European 1.97
textbooks on 1.1
tuberculosis and 3.50-.51
of women 7.6
Multiple myeloma 3.17
Multiple sclerosis, statistical series on 1.98
Mumps, statistical series on 3.2
    immunization data of 5.11
Muscular dystrophy, statistical series on 1.98
Muscular Dystrophy Association C.17
Musculosketal diseases, economic costs of 6.8
Myasthenia Gravis Foundation C.18
Myocardial infarction, cost changes in the treatment of 6.19

N

Natality 1.21-.22, 2.9-.10, 2.14
    statistical series on 1.89, 1.104, 7.2
National ALS Foundation C.19
National Association of the Deaf C.20
National Center for Child Abuse and Neglect C.21
National Electronic Injury Surveillance System, data from 3.7
National Foundation, March of Dimes C.23
National Health Survey (1935-36) 3.59

National Institute of Arthritis and Metabolic Diseases, Artificial Kidney-Chronic Uremia Program. National Dialysis Registry C.22
National League for Nursing 4.19, C.24
National Multiple Sclerosis Society C.25
National Prescription Audit 5.5a
National Safety Council C.26
National Sudden Infant Death Syndrome Foundation C.27
Nebraska
    health statistic sources of B.30
    regional depository library of D.26
Neoplasms, economic costs of 6.8
Nervous system, diseases of
    economic costs of 6.8
    number of cases and cost of care for 6.24
Netherlands, health care costs in 6.11
Neurological professions, manpower studies in 4.39
Neuropathy 3.26
Neurosurgery, manpower studies in 4.39
Nevada
    health statistic sources of B.31
    regional depository library of D.27
New Hampshire, health statistic sources of B.32
New Jersey
    health statistic sources of B.33
    regional depository libraries of D.28
New Mexico
    health statistic sources of B.34
    regional depository library of D.29-.30
New York
    health statistic sources of B.35
    regional depository library of D.31
North Carolina
    health statistic sources of B.36
    regional depository library of D.32

Subject Index

North Dakota
  health statistic sources of B.37
  regional depository library of D.33
Nosocomial infections, statistical series on 3.2
NTIS Statistical Data Reference Service B.91
Nuptiality. See Marriage
Nurse anesthetists, distribution and supply of 4.22
Nurses and nursing
  foreign graduates 4.29
  in hospitals 4.27-.28, 4.32
  manpower studies on 1.53, 4.9, 4.14, 4.17, 4.19, 4.23, 4.34, 4.38
  in physicians' offices 4.30
  statistical series on 1.89, 1.99A
Nursing education 4.14, 4.46
  bibliography on 1.53
  continuing education in 4.29
  costs of 6.13
  of foreign nurses 4.29
  statistical series on 1.99A
Nursing homes 4.4, 4.7
  directories to 4.3
  statistical series on 1.89, 1.99A, 1.112
  utilization studies of 5.8
Nutrition 3.43-.45
  among children 3.57a
  in underdeveloped countries 1.115
Nutritional diseases, economic costs of 6.8

O

Obesity, adult 3.44
Obstetrics 5.4
Occupational health and diseases 3.46-.47
  cancer 3.14
  indexes and abstracts to 1.63
  journals on A.22
  mortality statistics related to 2.16
Occupational therapists, manpower studies of 4.38
Oceania, cancer incidence in 3.25
Ocular disease 3.26
Ohio
  health statistic sources of B.38
  regional depository library of D.34

Oklahoma
  health statistic sources of B.39
  regional depository library of D.35
Optometrists, manpower studies of 4.20, 4.23, 4.38
Optometry
  education in 4.47
    costs of 6.13
  minorities in 4.9
  women in 4.9, 4.40
Oregon
  health statistic sources of B.40
  regional depository library of D.36
Orthopedic impairments 3.59
Osteopathic medicine
  education in 4.47
    costs of 6.13
  manpower studies of 4.10, 4.38
  minorities in 4.9
  women in 4.9, 4.40
Otitis media, cost changes in the treatment of 6.19
Otorhinolaryngology, manpower studies in 4.39
Outpatient services. See Ambulatory care

P

Pacific Ocean area. See Oceania
Pan-American Health Organization B.100
  bibliographical guide to the publications of 1.35
Paramedical personnel. See Allied health personnel
Parkinsonism, statistical series on 1.98
Pennsylvania
  health statistic sources of B.41
  regional depository library of D.37
Pertussis, immunization data for 5.11
Pharmaceuticals, cost and purchasing data on 5.5a-.5c, 6.16, 6.27
Pharmacists
  financial information on independent 6.13a

Subject Index

manpower studies on 4.23, 4.33, 4.38
Pharmacy
  education in 4.47
    costs of 6.13
  minorities in 4.9
  women in 4.9, 4.40
Physically handicapped. See Handicapped
Physicians
  blacks as 4.31
  fees and income of 6.21–.22, 6.26, 6.31
  foreigners as 4.44
  licensing of 1.101, 4.12
  manpower studies of 4.12, 4.16, 4.23, 4.38, 4.44
  statistical series on 1.89, 1.94
  utilization of 5.4, 5.8
  See also Family practitioners; Medical education; Medical specialties; types of doctors (e.g., Dentists; Osteopathic physicians)
Physician's assistants, education of 4.47
Pneumonia, cost changes in the treatment of 6.19
Podiatrists, manpower studies of 4.23
Podiatry
  education in 4.47
    costs of 6.13
  minorities in 4.9
  women in 4.9, 4.40
Poison Control Centers, directory of 1.19
Poisoning 3.9
  economic costs of 5.8
  indexes and abstracts on 1.63
Poliomyelitis, statistical series on 3.2
  immunization data of 5.11
Poor. See Low-income groups
Population and demographic characteristics 2.14, 3.59, 7.1–.15
  bibliographies on 1.50–.51, 1.54
  of blacks 7.11
  dictionaries and handbooks on 1.29
  guides to machine readable files on 1.80

of health professionals 4.36, 4.39
  indexes and abstracts on 1.61, 1.63, 1.70
  related to health facilities 4.1
  statistical series on 1.88, 1.99, 1.102, 1.104–.106, 1.109
  the aged 1.114
  underdeveloped countries 1.115
  textbooks on 1.4, 1.15
  of women 7.6, 7.13
  See also Census
Population Reference Bureau C.28
Pregnancy
  cost changes in medical care during 6.19
  economic costs of complications in 6.8
Prescriptions. See Pharmaceuticals
President's Committee on Mental Retardation B.93
Preventive medicine
  journals on A.28
  textbooks on 1.1–.2, 1.7, 1.14
Professional Activity Study–Medical Audit Program (PAS-MAP) 1.80b
Professional Standards Review Organization, directory of officials in 1.19a
Psittacosis, statistical series on 3.2
Psychiatric hospitals, admissions and residency period in 3.42
Psychiatrists, manpower studies of 4.15, 4.38
Psychiatry. See Mental health and illness
Public assistance programs 6.30
Public health
  bibliography on 1.43
  education in 4.42
  journals on A.6, A.29
  minorities in 4.9
  textbooks on 1.4, 1.14–.15
  women in 4.9, 4.40
Puerto Rico, health statistic sources of B.42

Subject Index

R

Rabies, statistical series on 3.2
Race. See Minority groups; names of minority groups (e.g., American Indians)
Rape 7.14
Rehabilitative services, for epileptics 3.38
Renal disease 3.26
Respiratory diseases
　economic costs of 6.8
　statistical series on 3.2
Reticulosarcoma 3.17
Rheumatism, statistical series on 1.98
Rh hemolytic disease, statistical series on 3.2
Rhode Island, health statistic sources of B.43
Romania, health care costs in 6.12
Rubella, statistical series on 3.2
　immunization data of 5.11
Rural health services, characteristics of 1.99

S

Salmonellosis, statistical series on 3.2
Samoa, American, health statistic sources of B.3
Sensory disorders, cases and costs of care for 6.24. See also Vision and hearing
Sex, statistics on. See Population and demographic characteristics
Sexually transmitted disease 3.53-.54
Shilgellosis, statistical series on 3.2
Sickle Cell Disease Foundation of Greater New York C.29
Skin diseases, economic aspects of 6.8
Smallpox, immunization data for 5.11
Smoking 3.48-.49
　among students 3.32
　among young men 3.37
　cancer and 3.14
　mortality rates and 2.15
Social security. See Insurance, social
Social welfare. See Public assistance programs

South Carolina, health statistic sources of B.44
South Dakota, health statistic sources of B.45
Spanish Americans, cancer among 3.16
Speech pathology, manpower studies in 4.39
State government
　checklist of publications of 1.34, 1.37
　directories to agencies of 1.19, 1.26, B.1-.55
　health care expenditures by 6.9
　See also names of states
Stroke, economic costs of 6.8
Students, drug abuse among 3.32. See also Medical education
Study of Nutritional Status of Preschool Children in the U.S. 3.57a
Surgery 5.4
　statistical series on 1.103
Sweden, health care costs in 6.12
Systems Development Corp., data files of 1.87, E.4

T

Teenagers. See Adolescents
Tennessee, health statistic sources of B.46
Ten-State Nutrition Survey 3.57a
Tetanus, immunization data for 5.11
Texas
　epidemiology of cancer in 3.16
　health statistic sources of B.47
　regional depository libraries of D.38-.39
Therapeutics, changes in the costs of 6.19
Tobacco. See Smoking
Traffic accidents. See Accidents and injuries
Trichinosis, statistical series on 3.2
Tropical medicine, journals on A.7
Tuberculosis 3.50-.52
　statistical series on 1.98

Subject Index

U

Ulcers, duodenal, costs changes in the treatment of 6.19
Underdeveloped countries, statistical series on 1.115
United Cerebral Palsy Association C.30
United Kingdom, health care costs in 6.11
United Nations B.101
  bibliographical guide to the publications of 1.35
U.S. Administration on Aging. National Clearinghouse on Aging B.78
U.S. Cancer Information Clearinghouse B.61
U.S. Center for Disease Control B.62
  National Clearinghouse for Smoking and Health B.77
U.S. Consumer Product Safety Commission. National Injury Information Clearinghouse B.65
U.S. Department of Commerce
  Bureau of the Census. Population Division B.60
  National Technical Information Service B.90
U.S. Department of Labor. Bureau of Labor Statistics B.59
  Occupational Safety and Health Statistics B.92
U.S. Government Printing Office. Superintendent of Documents B.98
U.S. Health Care Financing Administration. End-Stage Renal Disease Program B.68
U.S. Health Resources Administration 1.84
  Bureau of Health Manpower 1.40, B.57
  Bureau of Health Planning Methods and Technology 1.40, B.58
U.S. Health Services Administration. Maternal and Child Health Service B.71
U.S. Indian Health Service B.70
  hospitals of 5.12
U.S. National Center for Education Statistics B.73
U.S. National Center for Health Services Research, publications of 1.40
U.S. National Center for Health Statistics B.74
  publications of 1.39
  surveys of 3.57a
U.S. National Center for Health Statistics. Clearinghouse on Health Indexes B.63
U.S. National Clearinghouse for Alcohol Information B.75
U.S. National Clearinghouse on Drug Abuse, Alcohol, and Mental Health Information B.79
U.S. National Eye Institute B.80
U.S. National Health Planning Information Center B.81
  abstracting service of 1.65, 1.84
U.S. National Heart and Lung Institute B.82
U.S. National Institute for Arthritis, Metabolism and Digestive Diseases 3.27
  Diabetes Information Clearinghouse B.66
  Office of Scientific and Technical Reports B.83
U.S. National Institute of Child Health and Human Development B.84
U.S. National Institute of Dental Research. Dental Research Data Office B.85
U.S. National Institute of Mental Health B.86
  National Clearinghouse for Mental Health Information B.76
U.S. National Institute of Neurological and Communicative Disorders and Stroke B.87
U.S. National Institute on Drug Abuse. Division of Scientific and Program Information B.88
U.S. National Institutes of Health B.89, C.22

Subject Index

U.S. National Library of Medicine, data files of 1.84, E.3. See also Medical Literature and Analysis Retrieval System (MEDLARS)
U.S. Office for Maternal and Child Health Service. Bureau of Community Health Service B.56
U.S. Office of Cancer Communications. National Cancer Institute A.21, B.72
U.S. Office of Handicapped Individuals. Clearinghouse on the Handicapped B.64
U.S. Public Health Service B.94
U.S. Social Security Administration B.95
   Division of Disability Studies B.96
   Office of Research and Statistics B.97
Urban areas 7.7
Urbanization, infant and fetal mortality in 2.3
Utah
   health statistic sources of B.48
   regional depository library of D.40
Utah, University of. Eccles Health Sciences Library, data file of 1.86

V

Vaccination and immunization, statistical series on 1.116, 5.11
Venereal disease. See Sexually transmitted disease
Vermont, health statistic sources of B.49
Veterans
   costs of programs for 6.28
   mortality rates among smoking 2.15
Veterans hospitals, diagnosis in 3.60
Veterinary medicine 3.2
   education in 4.47
      costs of 6.13
   manpower studies in 4.23, 4.38
   minorities in 4.9
   women in 4.9, 4.40, 4.51

Violence, economic costs of 6.8
Virginia
   health statistic sources of B.50
   regional depository library of D.42
Virgin Islands, health statistic sources of B.51
Vision and hearing 3.55-.56, 3.59
   statistical series on 1.98
Vital statistics 2.1-.6
   bibliographies on 1.47, 1.51, 1.54, 1.57
   of blacks 7.11
   indexes and abstracts on 1.63, 1.68, 1.70-.71
   statistical series on 1.102, 1.106, 1.88-.117, 4.14
   textbooks on 1.4, 1.15
   See also individual statistics (e.g. Mortality)

W

Washington (state), health statistic sources of B.52
Washington, D.C., health statistic sources of B.10
Waterborne disease, statistical series on 3.2
West Virginia
   health statistic sources of B.53
   regional depository library of D.43
Wisconsin
   health statistic sources of B.54
   regional depository library of D.44
Women 7.6, 7.13
   in the health professions 4.9, 4.21, 4.25, 4.34, 4.51
   as dentists 4.11
   on medical faculties 4.18
   statistical series on 1.99A
   See also Nurses and nursing
Workman's compensation 6.28
   alcohol abuse and the cost of 6.6
World Health Organization, bibliographic guide to the publications of 1.35

Subject Index

World Health Organization. Distribution and Sales Service B.102

Wyoming
  health statistic sources of B.55
  regional depository library of D.45

X

X-rays, estimates of exposure to 5.9

Y

Youth. See Adolescents

Ref
Z
7553
M43
W444

DEC 17 1980